How to
by 1

How would you ....ply and
easily using a *fun* and *effective* method?

You *already* control your weight using your subconscious mind, like biofeedback. You program it *daily* to control your body weight— for better or for worse. Why not control it for the *better*? *Get slim and stay slim for good* by simply Thinking Thin.

"Debbie Johnson has compiled her knowledge & experience in a most thoughtful, insightful, and practical manner. Amongst the onslaught of weight-loss "hype", it is refreshing to have **How To Think Yourself Thin** to enthusiastically refer to friends, relatives, and patients alike."
— Dr. Steven Rotter, M.D., Center for Natural Medicine, Portland, OR

"I (now) have the incentive to select nutritious foods. It's easier to turn away from my old favorites— rich desserts, when I know it's by *my choice*, rather than because desserts are taboo. I like myself better as I am becoming. Thank you for your gift..."
— Joyce Franchett, CFP, Franchett Financial Services

"Results from dieting are far from satisfactory. A new approach must be found. Debbie Johnson takes you to the area of your being, the mind, the subconscious, the imagination, spiritual and feeling faculties — where the cause (and not the effect) is more likely to be found. A must for anyone who wants a thin body."
— Dr. Michael O'Grady, M.D., N.D.

How to Think Yourself Thin

Copyright © 1994 by Debbie Johnson

Cover and Interior Design: Michael Kronenberg,
MCA Presentation Services, Inc. Beaverton, Oregon
(503) 644-8906

Illustrations: Lee Wright, (503) 620-9873

Printed in the United States of America by:
BookCrafters, Chelsea, Michigan (313) 475-9145

ISBN
Library of Congress CIP Number Pending.

Published by Deborah Johnson Publishing,
7030 SW Canyon Crest Dr. #6
Portland, OR 97225
(503) 292-7657

Acknowledgments

There are so many thousands of people who have helped me get to this point in life and career, that to thank all of them would be impossible— but you know who you are. Here are a few who helped make this book, and the booklets previous to this, a reality.

I would like to extend my heartfelt thanks to the following people: For encouragement to start my publishing company— John Kulick and Lynn Heninger from Illuminated Way Publishing. And my friends Jackie Layke, Ed Ferrigan, Don Tousley, Gianeen Courrier, Terry Howard, Mark Morrison, Jocelyn Parrish, for either financial or moral support, and often both. For financial support, lots of ideas, and encouragement, my cousin Carol Polevoy. I'd also like to say how grateful I am to people like Bernie at Bernie's Supervalue in Minneapolis, Minnesota for being the first to try my books in his store. It's pretty amazing to have a "stranger" believe in you.

I'd like to thank the people who helped me put this book together from writing to editing to proofing— Zana Alexander, friend and editor; Harold Ware, John Eggan, Patrick Carroll, Michael Kronenberg (cover), and Lee Wright (illustrations).

A special thanks to my assistant Janel Nockleby who has done everything from proofing to keeping me sane and who has put up with me through all this, as well as waiting for paychecks when I was waiting for income!

A great deal of love and thanks goes to my mother for having set an example of an independent, strong person who went after what she wanted and always helped others along the way.

And last, but certainly the most important, I thank God for the love and guidance that is always present in my life.

—Debbie Johnson

Table of Contents

Introduction

I wrote *How to Think Yourself Thin* with love, to help you win the battle of the bulge for good. From age fifteen until just twelve years ago, I carried up to forty extra pounds of fat. My self-esteem was very low. It's not that I didn't have the willpower to diet. I lost weight on dozens of diets—only to regain it all back, and more, as soon as I started eating normally. Sound familiar?

My repeated failures at dieting were very damaging to my self-image. I didn't know that a good self-image was the secret key to achieving my ideal weight and sleek shape in a healthy, balanced way. I began to wonder if I would ever have the good fortune to be slim and trim. I felt very defensive—I even dumped one boyfriend who commented on my extra padding. What I didn't know, was that my thoughts were secretly perpetuating the fat— every minute of every day!

I finally gave up and decided, if God wants me this way, so be it! I learned to love and accept my rubenesque shape as though I were an artist, observing the curves and rounds as a sculpture—something in which I could see beauty. It made me relax, which allowed my subconscious to communicate a great idea to my conscious mind. I could try the same techniques I used to be successful in business! I had nothing to lose now (no pun intended). So what the heck?

My lifelong career in sales had taught me the effectiveness of positive imaging and feeling techniques for material success. I had thought myself better jobs, bigger contracts, nicer places to live, new furniture, and a great new car, so why not a new body?

I'll never forget the morning when I first began experimenting with the simple techniques in this book. I had just finished visualizing my sales goals for the day. The technique involved imagining my success for the day by telling myself I would sell an exact number of products during the next eight hours. I wondered if this same technique might work to control my physical self.

In sales, the first rule is to believe in your product. In this case, I had to believe in myself. I walked over to the mirror, looked into it and said with great conviction, "You look great, Debbie! Not only do you look great, you look a little thinner today!"

Immediately, I set aside some time each day to repeat my statement to myself and be grateful for whatever health and beauty I had. I became calmer about my weight, and realized that self-love and a new self-image could be the missing keys to my life-long problem with fat.

I had been dieting over and over again to change my self-image. Suddenly I asked myself, *How about changing that around? Change your self-image first, and maybe the healthiest means to reach and maintain the new you will follow.*

Over the coming months I crafted a new image of myself in my mind and ultimately lost forty pounds. Everything about my health, diet, and exercise subtly transformed—without any effort or willpower on my part. You see, I had discovered a great secret: Imagination beats willpower every time!

Thinking thin is a self-perpetuating phenomena which still continues to amaze me. Does it work? You bet it does. It's been twelve years since I lost the forty extra pounds—and I'm still lean and trim. The more I think I am thin, the more I eat, walk, talk, and act like a thin person. And the more I continue to act and automatically eat thin, the easier it is to maintain a comfortable, desirable weight. Thinking thin is also working easily and consistently for the many people who have attended my workshops over the years. You'll read about some of their stories in this book.

Here's the secret you'll learn to master: "I think like a thin person—because I am a thin person—because I think like a thin person!" These days, I am at the chicken-or-the-egg stage where I don't know which comes first. I just keep living life with the assumption that I am a thin person who can eat whatever she wants for health, whenever she wants—so I do!

I now find myself buying a favorite ice cream and leaving it in the freezer for days, because I don't have the time or inclination to eat it. Does that sound like someone with forty extra pounds who dieted on and off for years? I still love to eat and cook. I might bake a lemon meringue pie (my favorite) and eat it for breakfast, lunch, and dinner, and never gain a pound! Of course, I make it with a whole grain crust and honey for sweetener, —and I may eat extra salad for a few days afterward for balance. But the point is, I'm not forcing the issue through willpower. Thinking thin helps me be thin naturally.

As I mentioned, I have never regained the pounds that used to bounce back after every one of my strict, self-punishing diets. I threw out my scales. I find myself naturally drawn to different foods these days, without worrying about calories. I exercise lightly every day—and it's fun. I don't need to torture myself anymore!

Why? My new self-image, fueled by the creative power of imagination, makes being healthy easy and fun—without unnecessary struggle, strain, or forcing. I have learned how to talk to my subconscious—which only perceives images—and feed it a new picture of myself that gently drive all my actions to be healthy and consistent with being thin.

I know thinking thin can work for you too. I have never found anything for weight control more solid, secure, and permanent. Change your self-image and change your life!

Something You Can Do Now:

Begin this minute by imagining that you are svelte, strong, lean, and beautiful, just the way you would love to be. Make the image as realistic as you can, while fitting how you would most like to look. Describe this new image here, or in a journal, including the way you feel.

_____

_____

_____

_____

Doesn't it feel good to give that true, sleek self expression? In the chapters ahead, you will learn how to build on your thin, "key image" and hold the picture daily, for effortless, elegant weight control from the inside out.

About the Thinking Thin Exercises:

As you read, you'll discover dozens of simple exercises under the heading of "Something You Can Do Now." Most of them involve writing. Please take a moment to pick up a pencil and paper and set it next to this book. (There's a journal included in chapter eleven of this book, or you can begin your own journal in a notebook.) *This is important.* Writing is a very powerful tool for self-transformation. Writing makes your most secret and hopeful thoughts—your innermost self-image—tangible and real. You can see it there on the paper, in black and white. And as you write, you send powerful messages to your unconscious self, signaling it that you are ready to engage your creative energy for change—to heal your self-image and your life of excess weight.

How To Use This Book:

Here are some thoughts on how to use this book most efficiently and quickly if you are a busy person like me.

1. For most of you, reading this book from front to back is the best way to get a complete picture of how to think yourself thin. If you are as motivated as I am, however, and want to begin the process of thinking thin right away, you can also go directly to chapter five and choose one of the thinking thin exercises to begin using immediately as you read the rest of the book daily.

2. Chapter eleven includes a Thinking Thin Journal. You may use it all along, beginning immediately, or start your own personal journal. I do recommend keeping some sort of journal as you read this book, to make your personal process of thinking thin more real.

3. Chapter twelve is a review of the basic thinking thin principles. You can copy these pages and carry them in your purse or keep them in your desk at work for easy reference. This will help to keep you on track with your daily exercises.

4. For maximum efficiency in referring back to this book, I suggest highlighting the passages and exercises most pertinent to your personal situation.

5. I highly recommend *hanging on to this book* if you are using it at all, because it will keep you motivated and in tune with your thin self-image. Don't loan it to a friend while you are still in the first weeks of thinking thin. Tell her to get her own copy (through bookstores or 1-800-444-2524).

6. Most importantly—keep loving yourself, be patient with yourself, and have fun with this process!

Chapter 1

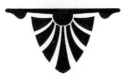

Why Can't I Lose Weight?

"The more I study the world, the more I am convinced of the inability of brute force to create anything durable."

—Napoleon I

As far as most people are concerned, diet is a four-letter word. I am no exception. It's not that I can't diet successfully. On the contrary, like millions of people, I have no problem dropping the pounds on a restricted diet. The difficulty lies in keeping the weight off once I quit dieting, just like many of you.

It all started when I was in high school (I won't tell you how long ago that was, because I am also thinking myself young!). A favorite pair of summer pants refused to fit the way they normally did. At the time, I didn't stop to wonder why all the rest of my clothes fit just fine. Instead, I screamed in panic. In my imagination, I just knew I was getting fat. My mother was successfully losing weight on the Weight Watchers program. Should I follow suit? I went on my very first diet and lost nothing. I didn't have much to lose at the time.

When my mother's best friend walked into the house one day with her world-renowned cherry-topped cheese-cake, the light struck me: I realized that my pants had simply *shrunk* in the dryer. I did not need to be on a diet! No, I needed to eat Babs's cheesecake and forget all this ridiculous stuff about being a certain size and shape.

That was the first time I ever engaged my negative imagination regarding weight. I started to wonder if I was fat. And like a bicyclist trying to avoid rocks on the road, I became so conscious of not hitting the rocks that I couldn't avoid them. The imagination works according to invariable laws—which you will discover in this book. What you image comes true. And what you imaged with strong feelings comes true even faster!

In college, my boyfriend looked at me funny one day as I bent over to pick something up. "Your tummy looks like it's sticking out," he commented. "I've never seen it do that before." Panic struck again, and I wasted not one second beginning a strict regime of cottage cheese and salad, the "skinniest" available dormitory food. Did it help the situation? No. On the contrary, it began my long slide into overweight unhappiness.

Over the next ten years I gained no less than forty extra pounds—all while on a continual merry-go-round of dieting. Looking back, I realize that I would not have gained the weight had I not been obsessed with the idea of being fat.

I remember feeling deprived when I would go on a special diet or fast. But as long as my willpower held out, I ignored the feeling, thinking how wonderful it would be to triumph over my excess padding (once again)!

When I got discouraged, I would pull out a greeting card with a cute, fuzzy teddy bear on the front that said, "I'm not fat, I'm just fluffy!" I'd tell myself that maybe I should just give up and enjoy being more huggable. But the idea didn't appeal to me as much as I would have liked. So I dieted some more, and fasted more—and the minute I started eating normally again, I gained back even more weight than I'd lost.

Ah, I can hear you now, asking, "Yes, but did you exercise?" Oh yes, religiously! I ran, swam, or danced three or four times a week. It didn't seem to make any difference. I moaned to my friends, "I can just smell food and gain weight! If I ate three whole meals a day I'd be as big as a house!"

I convinced myself that I was a walking sponge for every calorie that floated through the air. What I did not know was that I was actually giving my subconscious mind secret commands to increase my weight rather than reduce it. You see, I was trying to use willpower to lose weight. But my subconscious was responding much more readily to the fat images I was using to spur on my willpower. In fact, as you will learn through your own experience using the exercises in this book, imagination beats willpower every time. To really lose weight painlessly, it's much easier to "think yourself thin" using your imaginative powers.

The whole purpose of this book is to help you discover how your mind-body connection works. It's linked up through your subconscious. With the exercises in this book, you'll discover how to take a few simple steps to gain control of your eating habits, your all-important body image, and self-confidence. I truly believe I have found a missing link to help make your next diet your last—without worrying at all about what you eat.

It's all done with imagination. The subconscious responds directly to the image you hold of yourself. The subconscious does everything it can to make your actions—including what you eat, how much you exercise, and even your metabolic rate match your own self image. Willpower is no match for the imagination, because it does not have a direct link to the subconscious. Willpower is linked only to the conscious mind. To change the way you look forever, you need to tackle the secret pictures you're holding of yourself. How? It's fun! Beginning with the creative techniques in chapter five of this book you'll quickly learn how to replace those pictures with new ones. First, though, let's take a look at the pros and cons of traditional dieting.

Is There a Reason to Diet?

Joel Gurin shares the results of his dieting research in his article "Leaner, not Lighter" in *Psychology Today*, June 1989. "Two recent studies (Harvard Medical School and Stanford University) show absolutely no connection between calorie intake and body weight. The apparently obvious fact that fat people eat more than thin ones is simply not true." I know this to be a fact. It's the difference in what these people are imagining every day that contributes to being fat or thin.

Gurin mentions that some people have a "built-in tendency" to be overweight, but he also says "This doesn't mean it's futile to try to reduce...but the standard brute-force approach— simply making yourself eat fewer calories— is probably the least effective thing you can do."

Mr. Gurin reveals study results showing that both heavy and thin non-dieters eat remarkably the same. They both eat foods that they may not really need. Thin people, however, are much more sensitive to their body's signals about what and when to eat than chronic dieters, who often lose the sensitivity to their own natural eating guidance.

At one time I thought I was stuck with "fat cells," the wrong "setpoint," or some genetic weight condition. But when I decided I wasn't "stuck" with anything and started experimenting with thinking thin, my body began to change. Keep reading and you'll find you can change yours too!

Why Diets Don't Work

Every day, more people are struggling with their weight. Over half of all Americans are dieting or have dieted. Even though the diet industry raked in thirty-two billion dollars last year and is expected to exceed fifty billion by 1995, these diets aren't working. Upwards of 62 percent of all North Americans are clinically obese. That means they are twenty pounds or more over the (very generous) guidelines established by doctors for their height and bone size. Yet the only things becoming slimmer are the solutions! Why?

We are finally figuring out after all these years that diets don't work, due to the body's incredibly complex metabolic back-up systems. In fact, dieting may do you more harm than good. Here's how, according to many studies done by well-respected universities and experienced health professionals:

1. When the body is denied food it burns more muscle than fat, especially when the person dieting is not obese (twenty or more pounds overweight). Since muscle is the body's most metabolically active tissue, depleting it also lessens your ability to burn calories.

2. Calorie deprivation confuses your metabolism. In fact, each time you diet, your metabolism slows down and becomes more efficient to conserve calories. When you stop dieting, it may not bounce back to its former consumption levels. The added calories in your normal diet will likely be stored as fat—just in case that food famine you've been subjecting your body to returns!

3. The less you eat, the more likely you are to binge. If you restrict yourself to say, 800 calories a day, chances are you will be ravenous. Your body and your subconscious will do their utmost to accomplish one goal: get you to eat. You may start to wonder if you have any willpower at all—when in fact, willpower is simply no match for your survival mechanisms or your imagination. And believe me, at only 800 calories a day, your imagination will be constantly focused on the food you are missing.

Experienced dieters know that the more you imagine the food you are being deprived of, the more you want it. That's the real reason diets don't work. Your imagination will win out over willpower every time. Putting this fact to work in your favor is one of the secret keys to success you will learn about in this book.

Drastic calorie reductions can also lead to eating disorders. Evidence suggests a connection between low-calorie diets and disorders such as bulimia and anorexia. "Most people will credit a very low-calorie diet with their initial weight loss, but blame themselves (not the diet) for their subsequent weight gain," notes C. Wayne Callaway, M.D., director of the Center for Clinical Nutrition at George Washington University in Washington, D.C. This self-blaming cycle is very hard on your self-esteem.

Discouragement could cause you to begin binging and purging, slide into anorexia, or like most of us, simply give up in disgust at our lack of willpower. The side effects of this see-saw can be devastating, as you may well know, in terms of health and self-image.

So What Works?

Feeling totally confused about how to lose that extra weight? Take heart, that's why you're reading this book. It contains the tools you will need to (1) use your imagination to lose weight instead of beating yourself up with willpower; (2) create a new, loving self-image; (3) listen to your body's healthiest cues; and (4) naturally slip into the right food choices, exercise routines, and healthy thoughts that will create and sustain your ideal body weight.

How? Just keep reading. You will be given easy-to-use imaginative techniques that put you in charge of your weight and eating habits via the subconscious, the most powerful part of your mind. The subconscious controls your metabolism through the major glands and functions in the body. It also dictates how you feel about your body—another thing that will be changed for the better by the techniques in this book!

Before we begin to think thin, take a moment to write down your past experiences with diets (both positive and negative). This will give you a perspective on your dieting history so far:

_____

_____

If You Are Dieting Now or Plan to Go on a Diet

Considering the latest research, experts agree that life-style change is the only way to control your weight in a healthy manner. The diet you choose should meet the following criteria: (1) it should allow you at least 1200 calories a day, (2) the foods you eat should be very nutritious and fulfilling, and (3) with the help of this book, you should plan to make it your last diet!

If you feel you need to eat in a restricted manner as you work with the techniques in this book, be sure to also get the help of a doctor whom you are sure has the proper training to oversee diets. Recently, the American Medical Association recognized the importance of nutrition, and has made it a required topic in medical school.

A doctor with nutritional training is the best choice to oversee your diet. A few M.D.'s have proscribed extremely low-calorie regimens which have caused health problems for users—and even quite a few deaths (58 deaths among users of liquid protein products alone) in the past few years.

Problems associated with improperly supervised or very-low-calorie diets include:

1. Short-term complications such as dehydration, electrolyte imbalance, and increased uric acid concentrations.

2. Long-term complications such as severe ventricular arrhythmia, cholecystitis and pancreatitis.

3. For persons not severely overweight, large losses of lean mass can have disastrous consequences, including disturbance of cardiac function and damage to other organs.

Remember, you should try a really low-calorie diet only if your are at least 30 percent overweight, have received a recent medical examination and electrocardiogram with satisfactory results, and are free of contraindicating conditions, (such conditions include a recent myocardial infarction; a cardiac conduction disorder; a history of cerebrovascular, renal, or hepatic disease; cancer; type I diabetes; or significant psychiatric disturbance). All these restrictions do make one stop and think about dieting without an experienced doctor's supervision, don't they?

And don't expect diet weight loss to last. In researching articles on weight reduction, every one I read was very explicit regarding post-diet weight gain. It is assured in almost every case, and increasingly so with each additional diet. The reason? Survival.

The first function of the body is survival, naturally. If fewer calories are being consumed, the body reacts as if there is a famine going on. It has happened often enough in history. Why not now?

So what happens? The body's metabolism is slowed down to operate more efficiently. As a protective measure, more fat is stored against the unknown duration of food shortage! One third of all women polled who diet, diet about once a month. Dieting (famines) once a month, or even every six months would make for a pretty paranoid metabolism, don't you agree?

As many studies have shown, the body's lean mass (muscle) burns more fuel faster than fatty tissue. Dieters tend to lose muscle mass rather than fat, reducing their metabolic control hormones (located in the thyroid), so the body stores fat in greater amounts once the diet is ended (guarding against future "famines").

One study of laboratory animals showed that weight was lost two times slower and regained three times faster during the second round of yo-yo dieting than during the first round. It seems the animals were responding to lower calorie intake by using food more efficiently. The animals gained more fat after every diet, so even though body weight may have been lower, body fat soared—an unhealthy result for animals or humans. More fat lowers the operating speed of the body's metabolism, making it even easier to gain weight.

There are evidences of other unhealthy side effects to drastic calorie reduction. Diets may prove harmful to your immune system, and possibly increase susceptibility to breast cancer. Thus, the facts show that repetitive dieting not only doesn't work, but increases chances of weight gain and possible health hazards.

What about the Health Risks of Being Increasingly Overweight?

Though we may agree that diets don't work, we still need to find a solution to reaching a healthy weight. Most of us know there are health risks in being overweight. The most obvious are heart disease, high blood pressure, lessened ability to exercise, and of course negative psychological effects. The not-so-obvious risks are hypertension, some types of diabetes, and breast cancer (more likely after menopause).

Even moderately overweight women have a much greater risk of heart attack. A 5'4" woman who weighs between 150 and 171 pounds has an 80 percent greater chance of having a heart attack than a woman the same height who weighs only 125 pounds.

But there is still the double bind of trying to find a healthy solution to excess weight. Many people, instead of dieting, are gaining the self-discipline and responsibility to go on a lifelong program of eating lower-fat, lower-sugar, higher-fiber foods. This is great, but how do we know which foods are really best for us?

People today are demanding more and more diet foods. This means more and more low-calorie or no-calorie sweeteners, which have already been proven to be hazardous to our health, will be consumed. I happen to have a friend who lost her daughter to a food allergy. The autopsy revealed that she was hypersensitive to a no-calorie sweetener used in most diet sodas as well as in many other diet foods.

Many foods that are low in fat and sugar are also loaded with chemicals that may prove to be very unhealthy in the long run. Even the most sophisticated and disciplined dieters may not know how to really listen to their bodies in order to eat what they really need. Their notions of quality food may be arbitrary or ill-suited to their individual needs.

The solution seems elusive, but it can be found within these pages. And it works with just a few minutes of practice a day. This book will show you how to *know* what's best for you, as you rebuild your self-image. It will help you know just what to eat and when.

What about Exercise?

Exercise offers a partial solution to the weight-control dilemma. But people often approach it incorrectly, using willpower instead of imagination. Exercise doesn't seem to have any negative side effects as long as we use some common sense. Unfortunately, many people either overdo exercise, which can be counterproductive, or underdo it, which brings little or no benefit. These people need to let go of the mind and willpower and tune in to their body's real need for movement. Thinking thin helps you to do just this.

Becoming out of breath and red-faced is not necessary for health and fitness. As a matter of fact, that sort of stress on the body may be counterproductive. The harder and more suddenly you push your muscles, the more likely they are to raid your sugar (glucose) stores instead of the fat reserves. Moderate exercise will cause your muscles to use fat instead—the more desired result for weight control.

How Does One Know Exactly What Kind of Exercise to Do and When?

The problem with exercise is that we not only need to find the right kind of exercise, but we also have to know how to do it right, and how often. What kinds of exercise will burn the most fat? How high should our heart rate be? How much is too much, or too little?

And even if you know what kind of exercise you should be doing, you still need certain circumstances and characteristics to maintain a lifelong exercise regimen. Among other things you need time, discipline, motivation, desire, energy, commitment, and physical ability.

Don't get me wrong. I love to exercise, and sincerely believe in its benefits. If the beneficial results of exercise could be bottled and sold over the counter, someone would make billions!

But as with dieting, the limitations of willpower keep most people from exercising regularly and steadily. Just beginning an exercise program is not enough to up your health. If exercise is all you are relying on to lose weight, stopping after one month, skipping a week or two, then maybe going back after a year won't bring the results you want. Steady, regular exercise is required to develop and maintain an optimal metabolism that burns enough fuel so you can eat normally without putting weight back. So often, we run out of willpower to keep up a workable exercise routine day in and day out.

But again, imagination can be substituted for willpower with great results. It's not only more fun—it's a lot easier and more reliable than trying to force yourself to sweat

the pounds away. In the chapters ahead, you'll discover
how to harness your imagination for health. The key lies
in creating and holding your new, desired self-image.
Then the very best kinds of exercise for your particular
body and conditioning will come to you easily and naturally.

While not everyone will need to diet to lose weight,
you may not require exercise to get to the desired shape
and size of your new self-image. I enjoy light exercise as
part of my health maintenance, and for me it is truly fun.
I believe that is because it is driven by my subconscious,
which has now been programmed for optimal health,
youth, and happiness.

This book will provide imaginative exercises so you,
too, can make your subconscious your friend. Once you
do this for yourself, it becomes easier to find and use your
own tools for weight balance—ones that fit your particular life style, personality, and tastes.

A Word about Children and Young Adults

Statistics show our country's youth are heftier than
ever. Rates of obesity jumped up 54 percent from 1960
to 1980 among youngsters ages six to eleven, and 30
percent for adolescents between the ages of twelve and
seventeen.

Some parents are aware of the need to start regulating
their children's weight at a young age, but they go to ex-
tremes in restricting their children's diet. As we have
seen, this creates the least desirable effect, that of a slug-
gish metabolism and a rebellious will, as the young bodies
try to make up for the lack of food.

Articles on youth obesity usually suggest the same regimen for youth as for adults: low-fat, high-carbohydrate diets and exercise. However, if these measures have not been effective for adults, how can they be effective for children, who have even less control over what they eat due to parental and peer pressure?

Sixteen-year-old Christina decided she could do what I did and think herself thin. In one week she lost seven pounds! An eleven-year-old has lost twenty extra pounds in time to start school with clothes that are two sizes smaller than she wore last year.

Young people, particularly children, have a much more active and open imagination than older folks, because it has not been completely discouraged yet. I have seen them quickly win a new self-image, and thus a new body, using the very same methods outlined in this book. Joannie (eleven years old), who was in one of my "Think Thin" support groups, told me that after two weeks of thinking thin she was able to fit into clothes she had not been able to wear for two years!

The well-known fact that a high percentage of young girls are anorexic and bulimic is also cause for action. The techniques in *How to Think Yourself Thin* have helped young people improve their self-image and thus overcome eating disorders (see chapter five, How to Think Thin, working with younger children who have weight problems).

How Do Repetitive Weight-Reduction Attempts Affect Self-Image?

We have seen that health can be impaired by dieting, but that's not all. What about your self-image? How many people can emerge from the relentless torture of repetitive dieting feeling fearless, secure, and self-assured? Repeated failure, as any good psychologist will tell you, brings about fear. Fear induces lack of trust and confidence in oneself.

What is left to do on the diet scene? Keep punishing ourselves? We hope against hope that the "new" and "ultimate" diet programs will work. It does work, for awhile—then it abandons us. We struggle to maintain our new figure while beating ourselves up inside with guilt for eating all the food we had been denying ourselves (food that in fact the body may well need for good health.)

Many people who diet subconsciously feel they are being punished. I know I did. When I was at my fattest, if I looked sideways at something not on my diet, I felt as if everyone else in the room (mentally, if not verbally) was reprimanding me. As children, most of us were either punished or rewarded with food. "You'll go to your room without your dinner!" was a common threat. "Clean your plate and you'll get a nice dessert" was a bribe. "If you are good, you'll get an ice cream cone" was another. Is it any wonder people punish themselves with diets?

How helpful do you think punishment is to the self-image? The obvious answer is Not very. A good self-image is an absolute necessity to staying in optimum shape, in a healthy, balanced way.

We've been dieting to change our self-image. How about turning that around? Change the self-image first, and the proper means to reach and maintain the new body will follow! It has worked for me and for many others, so I know it can work for you too. I have never found anything for weight control more solid, secure and permanent. Change your self-image and change your life!

Begin right now by becoming aware of what your self-image is at this moment. Ask yourself how you feel about you, physically, and even in other ways (mentally, emotionally, spiritually). Write it in your journal:

_____

Now write in your journal what you would like your self-image to be if you could simply change it right now:

_____

The basic techniques to change your self-image and subconscious are in chapter five, Basic Exercises for Thinking Thin. Before we get to them, I want to share some of the whys, wherefores, and how-tos in order to make the subconscious mind work for you.

By they way, I put the key exercises for thinking thin in one place (chapter five) so you can easily refer to them again and again over the coming months. With the desire and commitment to change your self-image, you are well on the way to changing the total you. The only other requirement is doing a few simple imaginative exercises daily—a small gift of time and love to yourself in order to change your entire life. Ready to roll? Let's go—and remember to have fun!

Chapter 2

Who Really Controls Your Weight?

"Goals determine what you are going to be."
—Julius Irving

So, who controls your weight? You do, of course! You may not be completely delighted by what you have created, but be assured, you have created it for one reason or another and that means you can also change it. A part of you has always been in control and always will be. It's simply a matter of becoming conscious of how you've been in control, so you can start directing the process to your healthy benefit.

Many aware people have stumbled on this concept of self-image and how it affects their weight and health. John E. is a longtime owner of a very prosperous marketing consulting firm:

"The shape of my body is normally like my father's, *because I accepted that image long ago in my subconscious.* I haven't cared enough to replace it, so it's still there. Slightly overweight but not too badly, with the extra pounds in all the same places as my father's. I'm sure that's true of some other people, because parents are a dominant influence in our consciousness.

"But my body changes when I'm between relationships. I am interested in women a bit more, so I put more attention on my body image and tend to slim down. Then when I get involved in a relationship, the desire fades and I return to the old image

That tends to be a pattern with me.

"I have an older friend who is in great shape. He stands in front of a mirror every morning and has certain affirmations he makes about himself, and specifically his body, while looking in the mirror.

"Of course, I know imaging is important in business too. I am usually successful at what I do. If I am working on a project, I prepare for it, in such a way that I *see* or *visualize* myself being successful. Once I can see the route to success in my mind, in my imagination, then I proceed. That process is what I simply call planning!

"Most people think I'm a good planner. They see me plot objectives on a time line and prepare detailed strategies to achieve the objectives. But all planning really is for me is a way to see all the parts coming together. I know then what needs to be done, that it will work, and that in a sense, it *already is done*. This is what I call *knowing*.

John continues, "So the key ingredients I need to create something are: (1) a visual image of the outcome, (2) a written statement or plan about what I project will happen, and (3) a positive feeling about the project—which usually builds as I work on the first two ingredients. When these three modalities come together in an integrated way, that's *knowing.*

"A very good book on knowing and imagination is *The Flute of God* by Paul Twitchell. For instance, he points out that if you can't imagine yourself healthy, you won't be. A favorite principle of Paul Twitchell's is to reverse this approach—to assume the desired state of health, then ask yourself from this new, healthy viewpoint, 'What steps does it take to get here?'

"You have to really desire health and work with a certain feeling of conviction. Unfortunately, the media misuses these simple feeling and imagination techniques to get us to desire things we don't really need. Women's magazines, for instance, are always showing readers that they're supposed to be skinny. But if you apply this secret of imagining from the end to things you consciously want, it can put you in control of your life."

My own experience has shown me how important and powerful the imagination is, even when used negatively. Here's an example:

I remember once seeing a picture of a pig on someone's refrigerator. The person who owned the refrigerator wanted to lose weight. This person thought, logically enough, that the image of the pig would instill so much fear of becoming piggish that she'd be sure not to open the refrigerator door too often! I doubt that this tactic was very successful, though, because whatever we put our attention on is precisely what we become.

I experienced this phenomenon firsthand, as I mentioned in chapter one. The tragedy of the shrinking pants

and the boyfriend-and-the-belly scares was that both experiences, unknown to my naive consciousness, engaged
my negative imagination. I was unwittingly sending my
subconscious very clear commands for me to be bigger
and heavier (not fitting into my clothes) or to have a pot
belly.

How? In my fear of being fat, I constantly held the images of what I didn't want. Instead of warding off fatness,
these negative images manifested into physical form
within a few years of each scare. Think about it. If you
fear something, you tend to hold an image of it in your
mind, don't you? Fear is a very powerful stimulus to the
imagination. People instinctively acknowledge this when
they say to a fearful child, "Now, don't let your imagination run away with you!" It's a natural response to hold
an image of the things we fear most—but it's very destructive to our desired self-image.

In my fear of not fitting into my clothes or of having a
pot belly, I repeated key "fat" images in my mind hundreds, if not thousands, of times until they became a constant communication to my subconscious. My subconscious mind had no choice but to give me the results I was
imaging—even though I was imaging them unknowingly.

I am here to tell you that you don't have to make the
same mistakes I did. And if you already have, (as evidenced by the bathroom scale) be assured you can correct
your self-image with the techniques in this book, just as I
did.

Focus Only on What You Want— Because Whatever You Imagine Will Happen!

"Up until the age of thirty," Lisa told me, "I had no weight problem. In fact, I was extremely thin and underweight even though I ate like a horse! I could not get over a hundred pounds, no matter how I tried.

"Then I turned thirty and got a sit-down job. Did I ever begin to spread! I continued eating like I always had, yet I gained and gained. At one point I had major surgery, and after that I just couldn't lose the weight.

"I shot up over a hundred and fifty pounds. Going from not being able to get over a hundred pounds to being heavier than my slim husband just about killed me! It hurt to stand on my feet, and I wasn't comfortable. I knew I had to do something.

"I had been through a two-year period of dieting, and it was a really bad experience for me. I felt like I was starving to death the whole time! So I didn't want to diet again.

"I had never been disciplined enough to exercise, or to do anything repetitive for that matter. I wanted something really simple, so I didn't even bother trying any of the diets I read about, because I knew I wouldn't stick to it. I didn't want to change how I was eating. I was happy with my eating habits—I just wanted to lose weight!

"One day I happened to see your book, *How to Think Yourself Thin*, lying on somebody's couch. I became totally engrossed in it. I built a new self-image and began to keep a picture in my head of what I wanted to look like. That I can do. It's so easy! I don't have to change my diet; I don't have to go out and buy all this exercise equipment; I don't have to do anything. All I have to do is keep that picture clear and constant in my mind. Every time I think about myself, I just think about myself the way I want to look. If I look in the mirror and see myself the way I am physically, I just change the image in my head back to what I want to look like. And each time, the image in the mirror looks a little bit more like the image in my head.

"Thinking yourself thin is really easy and elegant! I can keep my new self-image going without willpower—because there's only one thing I have to remember—my fondest dream! I don't have to concentrate on sixteen things, just one! All I have to do is keep that picture the same. Every time I think about myself it has to be the same picture. When I first started, I had to decide what I really wanted to look like. I sat down and said to myself, I'd like to weigh so much and keep some well-rounded curves. I would look at women walking down the street and decide what I liked and wanted for myself. Then I put all my choices together to make a composite image of what I wanted to look like, and that's the image in my mind all the time.

"What happened first was that I came across a particular herbal tea which helped clean out my system. I didn't think anything of it at first. It was there, so I drank it. But one day I noticed a change. I was eating a little differently. It was a good change, and it was so natural I didn't even notice it. It went on that way, my desire for things I really didn't need to eat lessening day by day. It happened a little at a time.

"Then I realized that by keeping my new self-image constantly in my mind, the things I needed to help me manage my weight were coming into my life in a balanced, natural way. And it was easy to accept them. My husband and I went out and found an exercise bicycle at a yard sale, for instance, and now I am using it regularly. You have to understand, this is something I never thought I would do in a million years. But now it's just a natural flow. My new self-image is very powerful and is bringing healthy, natural changes into my life.

"Not only is my body slimming down (I have lost slowly, which is what I want, so it will stay off), but I have also quit chewing on my fingernails! That is a miracle in itself, because I have bit my nails all my life. I was born with my fingers in my mouth! I think holding my new self-image is a way to love myself more, and so I am now more relaxed about myself. I can also sit on my husband's lap again.. It's embarrassing when you're too heavy to do that!

"These positive changes all came about easily, just from holding that new image of myself. And I know it will just get better from here!"

Imagination Combined with Feeling Create Your Reality

Putting attention on anything with feeling draws it into our lives more quickly. Even though Jane, with her perpetual illness, did not consciously want to be sick, she became ill because she imagined she was sick and more importantly, *feared* being sick. The feeling of fear was an important key to influencing her subconscious.

Any feeling will help to create a driving force in the subconscious when using the focused imagination to effect a change.

If I were to be deathly afraid of getting fat again, that is exactly what would occur. I know I have to stay focused on the pleasant feeling of optimum health in order to stay thin and cancel out any fear of being overweight. It's not always easy to catch your thoughts and feelings in the act. Yet I've learned to be more afraid of being afraid, because I know what it will do: only cause problems that are unnecessary.

The more negative emotions, such as fear, anger, worry, upset, jealousy, etc. are those which cause the quickest response in the subconscious. Focusing attention on any image while feeling any of these emotions can bring about disastrous results. It's like putting a high powered, turbo-charged engine behind your thought!

An example of this would be a child's fear of falling off a bicycle and then doing so immediately (although children are generally fearless until we tell them about all the things they should be afraid of).

The reason the emotions work so quickly to bring about results is that they generally help to create a much more vivid image. If I ask you to picture a dog, for example, you may see a vague image of some sort of dog in your mind's eye.

What happens if I tell you to picture a vicious dog you had a bad experience with in the past? Has a dog ever scared you in some way? See how specific feelings and images snap into focus? Gently become aware of the feeling in your solar plexus (stomach area, just below the chest) as you think about the dog. You will probably feel some sort of fear or anxiety. Now, mentally erase that image and replace that image and feeling with a pleasant one—say of hugging someone you love. This is important because you want to stay clear of that sort of creation, even when it's just a memory exercise.

In fact, memories can be the most powerful influencers of the subconscious, because the feelings and images are right there in your image bank, ready to be called up. Beware of reminiscing, whether in thought, word, or action about past events that you would rather not re-create. (And *throw away* all those pictures of yourself—in your head and in your house—that look fat). Focus instead on what you are choosing to create with the exercises ahead.

Being Aware of Your Thoughts and Words Reveals to You the Control You Have

Being aware of how we think and talk not only helps us become more aware of who we are, but how much power we have over our lives. It's like becoming an observer and watching the process in order to get a feel for how it works. Try playing detective with yourself for a few days to see how your thoughts and statements make you feel and act.

Of course I have to watch my thoughts and words all the time too. I definitely pay for it when I slip up! But I just have to laugh at myself sometimes and that's the best way to stay "light" about working with your thoughts, feelings, and images. Guilt simply puts more feeling fuel behind your negative self-image and pushes it forward into your life even more.

We can be very positive thinkers about certain aspects of our lives and be totally the opposite about other aspects. This phenomenon constantly amazes me in my own life.

Focused Imagination Can Be a Detriment if Used Improperly

I have had a career in sales for most of my adult life and maybe even before that (does selling lemonade from a stand in front of the house count—or selling candy door-to-door for the Campfire Girls?). I learned by reading and listening to the masters of sales that visualizing success was the one factor that was absolutely essential to attaining it in any endeavor, whether it was sales or basketball!

My study of certain universal laws of life led me one step further. Visualizing was not enough. I had to imagine the successful outcome with all of my senses—smell, feeling, touch, and more. I will go in to more detail about this in Chapter three.

Even though I knew all about the power of the imagination, I neglected to apply it to my physical body and other areas of my life. I noticed I was constantly saying things to myself like, *I feel so fat!* and *I'm sure I'm gaining weight again,* or *I look like the Goodyear blimp.* Fear and anxiety, not to mention pure panic, combined with these statements to form very clear images. These images in turn cued my subconscious mind to put on the pounds.

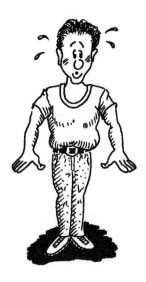

So of course I created more fat, more weight, and bigger dress sizes. I was in complete control of my weight, but I never would have guessed it. I kept giving my subconscious mind instructions to increase my weight via the vivid images with which I kept programming it.

Sometimes my negative imagination would run wild in another direction when I was having a bad day in my sales job. The feelings of failure would overcome me and I would be resigned to a "bomb out" day. It took a monumental effort to pull myself out of that feeling.

I could not always do it, so I would end up the loser. That's because thought plus feeling = image, and image = subconscious command. In this case the thought was:

It's obvious I'm not going to sell anything today. The feelings were remorse, guilt, and fear. The image was of myself at the end of the day feeling dejected and driving home discouraged and beaten, like a dog with its tail between its legs.

I suppose you can identify with this feeling from some time in your life. It's not much fun, but it can certainly be a learning experience. About the time I was driving home I would realize I had created the whole day by my initial attitudes.

I would then resolve to think positive the next day, even if I sold nothing. The idea was to stay on top of it, to know without a doubt that no matter what happened, I would be successful. I had put out the effort and it would come back to me. This is a universal principle, by the way, that you will learn how to put to use right away in Chapter five.

Joseph reads meters for a local utility company. He comments, "I get different routes every day. Sometimes I see it negatively. It may be a longer route, or there may be some things I don't like about it. When I think like that, the day becomes very long."

"If I turn that around and think, *There are some good people on this route I enjoy talking with*, I start to notice some of the little things that make it a nice day. My perspective on the route starts to change, and I notice thoughts such as: *It's not such a bad route after all.* Suddenly the day is going much better."

Joseph continues, "Another example of the power of thoughts happened to me recently. I needed a car, but I didn't see how I could afford it. So I tried thinking about it in a positive light. Every day when I drove to work, I kept saying aloud to myself, 'I'm driving in my new sporty car.' I kept a light, neutral feeling about it, telling myself I needed and deserved a new car. I decided not to sweat the details of how it would happen and where I would get the money. I saw and felt myself driving the car and was grateful for it.

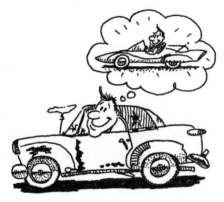

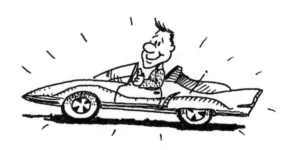

"Then I saw a dealer ad for the exact car I wanted—the same year, style and make I had been imagining. But when I went to take a look, I decided I couldn't afford it and let the matter drop. Over the next few days, the dealer called me back several times. Each time, he lowered the price over the phone until I went and bought it!

It was a full $3,000.00 less than what I thought I was go-
ing to have to pay!

"When I went to pick the car up, the manager just
looked at me and said, 'How'd you get the price so low?
I've never seen anyone get the price so low!' "

Something You Can Do Now:

Write a story here, or in your journal, about how your
imagination has worked for you in your career, a relationship, at school, with your family, in your health, or some
other achievement:

_____

_____

_____

_____

Write something you would like to have happen here,
or in your journal, that would be easy for you to imagine:

_____

_____

_____

_____

Teresa knows she can often have what she wants in
her life. Last time we spoke she told me, "I've come to
realize that you can really do whatever you want with
your life. Last time I moved I just visualized the kind of
house I wanted. I made it really clear in my mind. It took
awhile to get my new place, but when I got it, it was even
better than I expected.

"Often in my life I've had something happen because I
wanted it so bad I created it. You have to be careful with

this, because if you want something enough it is going to happen. Be sure you really want it."

Discovering the child within you that loves to imagine is one of the keys to seeing how you already control your life through your focused images and even certain actions. Children can teach us so much about the power of the imagination if we will only watch them and listen to them. Remember how you used to imagine what you would be when you grew up?

When I was a little girl, I wanted desperately to be a ballet dancer. I would find myself doing pirouettes and other ballet movements for which I had no name, pretending to be a ballerina extraordinaire. Then one day after school I heard another little girl say she was on her way to ballet class. My heart leapt at the thought that a second-grader could take ballet lessons. I'd never heard anything so wonderful in all my life.

I plucked up the courage at dinner that evening to ask my father if I could take ballet lessons. Evidently, we could not afford it, for he took one look at my dinner plate, with it's unfinished (shudder) lima beans and proclaimed, "Eat your lima beans, you'll be a ballerina!"

I wanted to be a dancer so badly that I believed him. Every time I ate lima beans during this time of little hope, I imagined they were somehow bringing me closer to my dream. Every lima bean was cleaned off my plate from then until I became a wizened pre-teen.

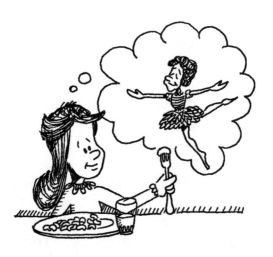

I finally gave up hope. By the time I got to college, I had forgotten my dream of being a dancer. Then my boyfriend began taking dance classes as one of his required Physical Education classes. I had long since forgotten my childhood dream, but he was having so much fun, I decided to try it.

Of course, I had no illusions of becoming a dancer, because such a career, I had heard, must begin as a child. Nonetheless, it sounded like a good way to get Physical Education credits. I was amazed at how wonderful I felt dancing, how exhilarating it was, how satisfying.

My non-professional dance career began then and there and I have been performing ever since, for hundreds and sometimes thousands of people at various gatherings. Dancing brings me one of the greatest experiences of bliss I have ever felt.

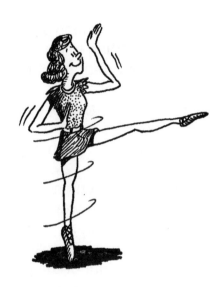

I realize now that my imagination brought me something even better than a professional dance career: a part time art-form I could enjoy thoroughly without the physical and financial stress so many professional dancers experience. I have the best of all worlds.

Something You Can Do Now:

Write here or in your journal something you imagined you would do in your future, and in fact did accomplish or see happen. It can be the smallest thing, like a vacation your family took, or a pen-pal you acquired.

Here is an exercise you can try to prove the strength of your own imagination. Say to yourself, or think to yourself, "I'm not going to eat that piece of chocolate cake."

What did you see or experience? Was it a piece of chocolate cake? If you have a vivid imagination like me, you probably saw yourself eating it too. How come, when you said, "I'm *not* going to eat that piece of chocolate cake?" Well, an important fact to note is that negative words such as "no, not, never, don't, shouldn't, or won't" are completely disregarded by the subconscious mind. Its supreme purpose is simply to receive the images that we feed it and make them happen in our lives.

If you kept repeating the sentence, "I will not eat that piece of chocolate cake", you would soon feel driven to eat it. Eat the cake, and think to yourself, "Everything I eat turns to energy." By the same token, the person who continually looks at her picture of the pig, might internalize some part of the pig's tendency to overeat.

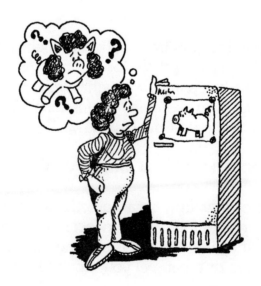

Want to reverse the process? It's easy...try this exercise: Think to yourself: I'm healthy, slim , and strong, and I can eat whatever I want!

What did you imagine? By replacing the image, you reversed the process. In fact, you have actually given your subconscious mind a command in the form of images. Now you will eat only what is good for you most of the time, enough of the time to keep you healthy, and when you feel like eating chocolate cake, let yourself eat it and enjoy it, and know you will balance it just fine. In chapter four we will talk more about the language of the subconscious and how it works.

For now, here is an exercise to begin your very important next step in the process of thinking thin:

Something You Can Do Now:

Imagine right now that you are svelte, strong, lean and beautiful, just the way you would love to be. Make the image as realistic as you can, while fitting how you would most like to look.

Sherry claims she was very homely as a child. She kept looking at a photo of a famous movie star who was just a little older than she was at the time. She kept imagining that she looked this way, kept telling herself she looked this way, and kept believing that she would become the pretty person she knew she could be. She is now, in my estimation, much more beautiful than that movie star, inside and out.

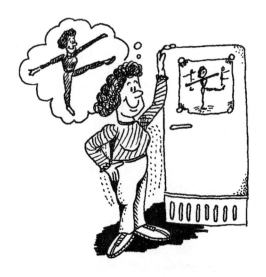

Feel how it feels to be the way you want to be. Get into the sensation of being already successful in having achieved your goal. What kind of emotions does it bring forth? Write them here or in your journal:

_____

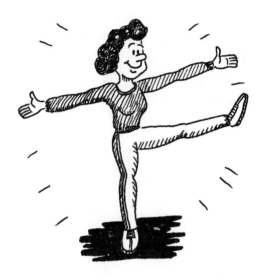

Now imagine yourself performing some activity in your new body. What are you now thinking about yourself? How do you feel? Write it here or in your journal:

_____

How does your new self affect your relationships with others? (still thinking from your end goal of the "new you"):

_____

As you go about your day, identify some of the things that happen because of your imagination. It's easy to spot after a while. Once it becomes a habit, you see that your life isn't such a mystery anymore. As you become sensitive to your own and other's thoughts and words, a feeling of being in control of your own life will begin to grow. It is a freedom beyond words!

Focusing on the *goal* you want to achieve, rather than any limits or roadblocks you may perceive, is the sure way to success in any endeavor from sports to business to controlling your body weight. You can be as creative as you like with your imagination.

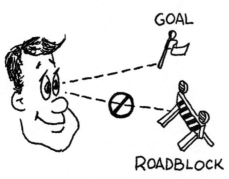

Every sentient being has a subconscious mind. But that being is much more than mind; it is a divine Soul, able to consciously choose Its experiences. Techniques will be given in Chapter 5 to move beyond the conscious and subconscious mind as well as outer influences such as other people's words and thoughts and society's images.

No one of us can ever be perfect. But each of us can reach for perfection. In so doing, we unfold in our consciousness, wisdom, and love of life.

Chapter 3

How I Discovered the Secret of Thinking Thin

"If your ship doesn't come in, swim out to it!"
—Jonathan Winters

Thinking thin was not something I did naturally. It was an idea that came to me after many years of studying and applying certain principles learned in business and in my spiritual studies. In this chapter I'll show you how these principles of self-image and imagination worked for me in sales and how I then applied them to changing my body weight and image.

My years of experience in sales has taught me that you have to do a lot more than just *think* positively. You also have to:

1) Hold a very *good self-image.*
2) Set a realistic *goal.*
3) *Write* the goal down.
4) Assign a *deadline* to achieve your goal.
5) *Visualize in detail* the goal being fulfilled; i.e., see the contracts being signed and the customer writing a check.

6) *Imagine* what it *feels* like when your goal is met: the gratitude

and joy, the state of beingness that embodies your goal fulfilled..

7) *Act as if* the goal is already an established fact.

8) *Persist* in all of the above!

9) *Create* a plan and *act* to achieve it.

Whatever sales goal I imagined using this formula was achieved. If I did not reach the desired outcome, it was almost always because I let fear, worry, or insecurity creep in and take over my imagination. The simple recipe of positive feelings such as enthusiasm, excitement, gratitude, or inner peace and contentment along with the visualization of the goal caused it to come about.

How I Learned to Think Thin

The methods of positive imaging and feeling combined with assuming the goal fulfilled worked for me in sales and other business endeavors, but I had not yet made the connection to using them to manage my body weight and shape. After years of dieting and going back to eating what I thought was a very modest amount of food carefully chosen, I was still struggling with about thirty pounds of extra weight.

Then one morning as I finished visualizing my sales goals for the day, I began to wonder if I could "think myself thin" using all the positive imaging and feeling techniques I had learned. After all, I had thought myself better jobs, bigger contracts, better places to live, new furniture, and a great new car—why not a new body, too?

I walked over to the mirror, looked into it and said with great conviction to myself, "You look great, Debbie. Not only do you look great, you look a little thinner today!"

And do you know what? I felt a little thinner. I decided from that moment on, I would feed myself positive images to become the way I wanted to be. What could it hurt? I certainly didn't have anything to lose, except some fat!

In this chapter I will show you how I applied each of the principles which brought me success in sales to thinking thin.

Self Acceptance Was an Absolutely Vital Foundation

The word "sales-person" has a very negative connotation to most people and I was no exception. In my own mind, I'd decided that I'd never choose most salespeople for close friends or even acquaintances.

I was introduced to sales via a nutritional product I bought from a friend. It was a very good product and I felt like it could help a lot of people, but I never even thought about selling it. My friend convinced me to go to a meeting with her about selling this product by telling me not to think of it as selling, but sharing something I believed in.

This key concept formed the foundation for my success in sales. Seeing this potential career in such a positive light, and more importantly, myself as a helpful salesperson providing a valuable service, formed the basis of my decision to try selling. My self-image had been the

only thing holding me back from a successful future in
sales. Now I had the freedom to be what I was destined
to be; someone who could *share* products and services
that would enhance the quality of life for others.

Still, other people called me a salesperson, and somehow I had to come to terms with the fact that my liveli-
hood was best made in sales and I was a salesperson, no
matter what other fancy names I might be given (consultant, marketing representative, account executive, etc.).
How could I gain the respect of the customer if I was a
"salesperson", I wondered.

The answer for me was to go back to the idea of sharing, and more importantly, being of service. The key
word, image and idea for me was service. It was sincere
and true, and I knew that almost anyone I spoke with
would sense my goodwill in their hearts.

The instant I walked in the door, I wanted my customer
to know I was there in their best interest. I decided to
keep this in mind as much as possible during my work
day. As I approached an appointment or talked with a
potential client, I would say to myself, *"I am here to be of*
service, in a way that is best for all concerned."

Confidence in my product was also a very necessary
ingredient to service, and therefore to success. I studied
all the facts about my own product versus the
competition's products. I had to know I was representing
the best.

I would write down everything that made my product
unique and better than similar products on the market.
Before I consented to work for a company, I interviewed

their customers to see what they liked about the company's products. These satisfied customers gave me the conviction to share the benefits of the product with others.

Once my whole being radiated belief in myself and my product, I became a truly successful representative for it, and was generally the top salesperson in the company.

As sales went up due to this building of confidence, my self-esteem continued to rise and I was able to get almost any job I wanted in sales. It was a matter of choosing exactly what I wanted to do and going after a job.

My confidence on the job became pretty solid. There were situations that shook me, but I always looked back at my abilities and my intentions to serve and it carried me through the rough times.

Once I was selling insulation door to door on a special government program to help people conserve energy. The customer thought I was working for the local utility company, which almost everyone was unhappy with at the time. He tore into me before I got two words out. I just stood there and listened, trying to empathize with what he must be feeling. I let him get it all out of his system, then told him I certainly agreed with some of his views.

To make a long story short, he ended up insulating his entire home through our program and sent me to see some of his neighbors as well! The self-confidence I had built allowed me to successfully weather little storms like this, whereas without it I would have turned tail and run cowering in the opposite direction!

Self-esteem, Self-acceptance, and Self-love Came First in Thinking Thin Too

The first step to thinking myself thin was belief in my product. This meant accepting myself for who I was! I immediately set aside some time each day to notice and be grateful for the health and beauty I had.

Why? Because, just as in sales, I had to radiate confidence in my product. In order for to be calm and clear-headed about my experiment, I also had to be neutral about the outcome of my life-changing efforts. Any panic or anxiousness would fuel my subconscious with negative images. I became calmer about my weight, not even knowing I was doing it, when I said to myself and to God, *"If this is the way you want me, so be it."*

"Belief in the product" meant identifying the unique qualities I have that no one else has. I worked at seeing the beauty that was already there, and accepting everything else as a part of who I needed to be at this time in my life.

Setting Goals is Absolutely Vital

A ship without a course goes nowhere. That is just about where I went when I had no goals. Goals are motivators, and they also work with the subconscious mind to steer a course for success by creating a destination out of an image.

On the job, I learned to set daily, monthly, and yearly goals for myself. I tried to strike a balance between numbers that were both challenging and reachable.

My spiritual studies have been a tremendous boost in learning the spiritual or subtler laws of life and how to apply them to everyday goals. One of the key spiritual laws I applied is called the Law of Cause and Effect. Ralph Waldo Emerson called this the Law of Compensation. The Bible tells us that we reap what we sow.

This law is very exacting. It is summed up in the scientific postulate: For every action, there is an equal and opposite reaction. In my experiment, it meant that if I programmed the subconscious in a certain way, it would respond by manifesting the images I fed it.

The next piece of the puzzle was gained in a business workshop I attended. Here I learned the importance of writing down my goals and assigning deadlines to them. The instructor told of a study that showed the importance of actually writing down goals, versus merely thinking about them.

In the study, the first group of people were instructed to make up a goal for themselves, think about it, and work toward it each day. A second group was given the same assignment, with the additional instruction to write their goal down on paper. The group that wrote down their goals was 100 times more effective at realizing their goals over the group that did not!

After I heard that story, I began to write down all my goals, and assign a date for their attainment (which was also stressed in the workshop). I recorded my sales goals for the month and the amount of money I wanted to make. I also included a list of things I wanted to obtain by the end of the month, such as a new piece of furniture, or some article of clothing.

It absolutely amazed me at how precisely this goal-setting process worked. Even when I did not go out and buy what I had written down, someone would often give it to me!

Another way I used cause-and-effect goal-setting was to find a new apartment or condominium. I would make a list of every single detail I could think of, such as rent amount, location, size of rooms, facilities and amenities, parking, noise level, quality, etc. This helped me form a detailed, real image of what I wanted to create. The only time I was ever disappointed was when I left out an important detail, like how big the bathroom should be!

Setting Some Kind of Goal is Important for Weight Control Too

I found myself thinking about what kind of body I would really like to have. I mean, if I was going to change anything about my body, why not change everything I could think of? I decided I wanted to be healthy, somewhat muscular (I was tired of being a wimp) and lean. I added the caveat that I didn't want to be overly muscular, like a body builder, just strong and athletic-looking.

My desire for strength reflected a need for inner strength, which is a common need in people who are overweight.

I called my new picture of myself my "key image." It was exactly how I saw myself looking when I reached my desired goal. I imagined a feeling of confidence and the strength of a good dancer as I settled into this new body image.

I didn't set a goal for weight in pounds, as I felt that would get in the way. Of greater importance was the health of my body, not the exact weight, and I had a clear image of how my healthy body would look, feel, and act.

I Learned to Focus on the Goal Using My Imagination

Learning about how the subconscious mind works was an interesting process for me. The best advice I was given was in regard to the use of negative words. One of my sales trainers was the Vice President of Marketing for my company and a very well-read, experienced marketing professional. He explained something to us that has always stuck with me. I am sure it has been an important part of whatever success I have attained in sales.

His secret? The subconscious mind does not hear negatives. In other words, if you say, *"I am not going to do that again!,"* your subconscious hears, *"I am going to do that again."* This is because your subconscious only deals in images. It sees the image created by the words, *not* the words themselves.

Say to yourself right now, "I will *not* think of chocolate cake." What do you immediately think of? I rest my case. This principle put the fear of God into me about how I spoke to myself. Instead of saying, "I'm not going to bomb out today." or something to that effect, I would keep reminding myself of my goal image by saying, "I'm going to sell twenty of these by noon," or "I can feel this is going to be a great day!" That kind of self-talk always made me successful, even if it took an extra day for the subconscious command to kick in.

Being positive all the time is impossible, I soon discovered. Learning how to be positive most of the time was a challenge too, but I knew I could do it with persistence. I heard someone say that if you do anything for 28 days in a row it becomes a habit.

I believed that and decided to try it with my thoughts. It worked fairly well, but again, was not necessarily easy. Changing thought patterns takes time and patience with oneself. If you want this to work for you too, you must be persistent and give it lots of time.

Another powerful principle of focused imagination has to do with replacing old images or thoughts with new ones. In my spiritual studies I read that in order to get rid of an old habit or thought, I had to replace it with something new. An common example of this is chewing gum or breathing deeply instead of smoking a cigarette when one is trying kick the habit. I found a joyful freedom in making a conscious choice of what to replace my fat images with.

I'd already replaced old negative thought patterns with new ones in my career and financial life. Sometimes I would even pencil in the amount of money I wanted to see in my bank account that month in my checkbook register. When the real amount presented itself, I used pen to write over the figure in my account. Seeing the larger penciled in amount every time I opened my checkbook gave me a boost.

Sales also taught me to work with the customer's imagination to find out if they were really serious about buying my product, or if they liked the particular model you were showing them. For example, with computer sales I would ask the customer where they might put the computer in their home. I could see the wheels turning in their minds, as they pointed mental fingers at corners and cabinets.

When they would say, "Oh, I'll just take out those shelves over there and buy a stand for here..." etc., I would know they had just bought a computer. Whether they bought the computer from me was sometimes another story, but at least I got them to take the mental leap into accepting something greater in their lives. I used the same technique asking myself, *"What kinds of clothes are you going to wear when you're slim?"* And, *"Don't you feel good about eating?"* More about this later.

Focused Imagination is the Heart of Thinking Thin

One of the first things I did when I began thinking thin was emphasize the importance and high position of my imagination as the controlling factor in my life. I threw out my scales! I refused to weigh myself thereafter. Who needed the fear the scales instilled?

When I went to the doctor for a checkup, I almost told the nurse to go take a hike when she wanted to weigh me. She then had the nerve to tell me I needed to drop a few pounds! In whose book? I thought, resentfully. I was feeling a little defensive and proud of myself for losing fifteen pounds so far. After all, I was well on the way to a new me, no matter how it looked to her or anyone else.

Weight was coming off at a slow, steady, and healthy rate that was right for me, and I was enjoying life. I knew

if I just kept my imagination glued to my key image with a
sure confidence, I would be slim before I knew it!

Radiating Confidence Was a Vital Ingredient

Dennis Waitly, author of "The Psychology of Winning", gives wonderful lectures, one of which I was fortunate enough to attend. He works with a wide range of clients—from astronauts to Congress people and top ex-
ecutives.

One concept from his talk really stuck with me. It was
to accept compliments gracefully, even knowingly. This
was a most effective means of boosting my self-confidence in all areas of my life. How many times have you
complimented someone on their hair and heard them re-
ply, "Oh, it's such a mess today, I don't know how you
can think that!"? Most people are simply too caught up
in a negative self-image to accept that someone else
might think they look great.

I began to notice how difficult it was for me to accept
compliments and just say "Thank You." You know how it
sort of gets caught in your throat? Especially if you feel
the compliment is undeserved. I *made* myself say
"Thank You" to *every* compliment and then *shut up*. It
was amazing to watch my self-image transform over time.
I actually began to *believe* what people were saying about
me!

Becoming my own health authority was the next step
to radiating healthy confidence. In sales, I had already
decided to write my own script in the play of life instead
of letting others write it for me. For example, in a sales

meeting, I would announce my goals with unshakable be-lief. Even though they were higher than everyone else's and I got a few raised eyebrows, I would stand my ground. Most of the time, I proceeded to reach the goal and win salesperson of the month.

Not only did I meet my sales goals, I accomplished them in a manner that suited my ethics, honesty and lifestyle. Even though everyone else in my insulation company thought they had to call on people during dinnertime when they were at home, I refused to inter-rupt people's dinner.

I decided I would find my clients at home during the day and make appointments to meet with the spouse at night, working Saturdays if necessary to catch other people at home. Working the "least optimum" sales hours, I was the top salesperson in that company for three years!

Radiating Confidence Works With Weight Management

As I mentioned earlier, the most important thing I learned from Dennis Waitly was how to accept a compli-ment. It boosted my self-confidence at a crucial point in my crusade to think thin. People started noticing my weight loss and complimenting me on it left and right.

I accepted every compliment with a "Thank you" and believed what the person said, deciding to view myself as objectively as possible. I stood up straight and proud. I wore clothes I felt comfortable in. On dates, I chose clothes that flattered my body's good points rather than emphasizing its weaknesses. I made sure the clothes did not pinch or make me feel fat! I chose to see myself as beautiful, and others started seeing me that way too.

I knew that how I viewed myself was reflected in my presentation of myself and in my body language. People complimented me when I chose to think of myself in a favorable light.

Acting As If the Goal is a Reality Right Now Makes it Come True Faster

A little-known, seldom-taught phenomenon of the subconscious mind was given me through my spiritual studies. You can see it in those who are successful in sports, business, or any endeavor in life. This secret is to "act as if" the goal has already been met.

For example, you may often hear Olympic gold-medal winners explain their victory in these terms: "I never even thought about failing", or "I just saw myself winning, I wouldn't accept anything else."

I applied this principle to get to get the successful-looking car I needed. I had been driving a small, modest economy car that looked nice, was new and got me where I wanted to go. The only drawback was that it was not the image I needed or wanted to create as a marketing consultant, the role to which I was aspiring. I kept imagining I owned as a Mercedes Benz, or some other impressive vehicle. I would imagine I was driving my new car as I cruised down the highway.

When I would talk about the car I still had, mentioning the model, people would often say, "Oh, I thought your car was a Mercedes or something." Their reactions confirmed I was doing a good job of assuming the wish fulfilled. One day after giving a goal-setting workshop, a client walked out to my car with me and did a double take. He said, "Gosh, I thought you'd be driving a Rolls Royce!"

A few months later I had the opportunity to buy a nearly new Mercedes at a very reasonable price. Once the opportunity presented itself, it did not appeal to me as much as a brand new model sports car that was very luxurious for the same amount of money I would have spent on the Mercedes. I bought the sports car, but the point is, I had the opportunity to easily obtain what I originally wanted because I was able to hold the image of it. It also showed me that I could change my mind for something even better!

In Thinking Thin I Also Acted As If the Goal Had Already Been Reached

I knew I was on the right track with thinking thin when a friend commented on a dance performance during the beginning stages of my process. She said, "I never thought someone with your weight would look that good dancing up there, but you looked wonderful!" Of course I was taken aback by her comment, since I wasn't viewing myself as fat any longer. But I also noted her ability to see beauty in the dance and accept me as I was accepting myself. It was as though she was seeing the "new me" that I was projecting by my strong inner images. This made me feel that my "acting as if" was beginning to gell.

Not weighing myself helped boost my spirits tremendously. It gave me the freedom to think of myself as truly thin. Even though I had some setbacks when people commented on my heaviness, I stuck to my inner image like glue and kept the feeling of knowing I was already there!

Persistence Meant Never Giving Up, No Matter What Happened

Keeping loving attention on my goal in the face of failure was not easy. Inspirational books on positive thinking and success were very helpful to me when I needed to break through some heavy barriers or cross a few muddy trenches in the subconscious. Success-oriented business magazines always seemed to have something encouraging to read and were helpful in bolstering my persistence.

Persistence always paid off. When I was working on the insulation program with large condominium complexes, I held an image of a check for $20,000 made out to me. I did not know which contracts would come through, nor did I imagine any specific contract coming through (as that would be interfering with the spiritual freedom of other individuals). But, I did keep visualizing this large amount. I knew it was possible to earn it, even if it came in smaller amounts that added up to $20,000.

All summer I waited and nothing came through. I kept persisting. Still nothing. Finally Fall came and the money started rolling in. By January I had earned $35,000 with ease! It was the first time in my life I had ever been able to keep my imagination focused with such persistence and on something that seemed impossible.

After I earned this money I planned a vacation in Hawaii. I realized a celebration was an important way to acknowledge my completion of the goal. I had been imagining myself in Hawaii for years. Every time I went to the beach, I'd close my eyes and imagine palm trees swaying on a beach in Hawaii. When I heard music with waterfalls in it, I would close my eyes and be near a waterfall in Hawaii. I had imagined Hawaii so well that after taking a cruise of the Hawaiian islands, I ended up moving there for five months!

Persistence has always paid off in sales, whether it be working longer hours to make my goals, trying harder to reach the right person on the phone, or simply keeping my attention riveted to the goal without compromise. It is the one ingredient sales veterans claim as the absolute secret to success.

Persistence Meant Never Giving Up On My Key Image of Myself

No matter what I saw, heard, read, dreamed or felt, I constantly looked for ways in which I was succeeding. I constantly told myself I was reaching my goal. For example, whenever I was about to walk by a mirror, I would expect to look great and say aloud to myself, "I am going to look thinner." Then when I got in front of the mirror, I would say to myself, "I look thinner, I'm getting thinner every day"—even when I did not feel like it!

At one point I started gaining more weight, even after I had been seeing myself thin for awhile and telling myself I was getting thinner. My old negative thoughts were still having some effect because there is sometimes a time lapse until the new positive thoughts take over. I just persisted in my "thin" thoughts that much more. I knew from sales that the time to keep going was when I least felt like it. *That was when real progress seemed to be made.* I also knew from the stories of many successful people that when everything seems to be going against you, that is the *most important* time to keep going! It is truly a test of our inner strength—and always a good strengthener to meet the challenge. There's a reason why people say, "It's always darkest just before the dawn!"

When I heard that Abraham Lincoln lost sixteen elections before he won the election for President of the United States, I felt I had faced nothing compared to him, or to other men and women who have climbed impossible mountains. I was thoroughly determined to make my life what I wanted and to make it worthwhile!

How Can I Be of Service?

Service means being of assistance to others. How did that help me in sales? I felt it was crucial to establish the client's trust in my company and me by providing whatever help I could during his or her decision-making process. That sometimes meant tracking down answers to obscure questions, making special phone calls for referrals, obtaining extra literature, or sending out a copy of some relevant article. I held a feeling of wanting to truly do what was truly right and best for the customer, within the framework of my knowledge, ability, and the company I worked for.

More importantly, being of service means coming from the heart—doing everything you do with love. I knew the customer would perceive this love and sincerity. It also meant living my spiritual beliefs and remaining neutral about the outcome of any particular sale. I projected love and respect for my fellow being whether she bought something from me or not. That attitude, when I could hold it, created much more success for me than I would have otherwise realized.

Being of Service Takes Attention Off Me and My "Problem"

I knew it would be selfish to focus all my attention on creating a new image for myself without being of service to others, I tried to see how my new body would be a ve-hicle of service to God and to others. I knew I would be healthier, thus able to be of greater service with more en-ergy. I would also feel better about myself, which would help me appreciate others more.

Perhaps I would serve as an example for someone else who shared my frustrations with weight control. Inciden-tally, that is my sole motivation for sharing the techniques of thinking thin with you! Every day, I looked for old atti-tudes and beliefs to replace with images and actions of service, such as working in my community or being kind to someone on the job.

Benefit From My Years in "The School of Hard Knocks"

It took me a long time to amass these basic principles through my business and spiritual studies. You can take advantage of my long process to streamline your own thinking thin process, which will be described step-by-step in this book.

Success can be yours by following the road map in this book and the basic exercises outlined in chapter five. But first, I'll explain why the process works, so your mind will be happily convinced to move forward without reserva-tion.

Chapter 4

Why Thinking Thin Works

"Imagination is more important than knowledge."
—Albert Einstein

Understanding why and how these methods work will convince your mind of the logic in trying them. This chapter provides important information on the whys and wherefores of thinking thin so your mind will understand it.

I believe this weight management method will work best and fastest when you consciously grasp the mechanics behind it. The mind is a very strong force in your life, so giving it straightforward information to mull over is wise. So what are the dynamics of thinking thin?

The Subconscious Mind Controls All the Major Glands and Functions in the Body

Almost any doctor will tell you that the mind and body are very much connected. How many times have you read or heard about new research concerning the mind or emotions influencing diseases like cancer or arthritis in a positive or negative manner, depending on the patient's attitude?

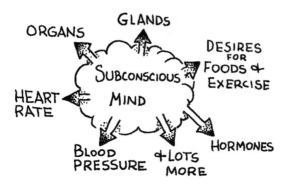

The subconscious mind in particular controls the body twenty-four hours a day, even while you are asleep. The conscious mind commands your body to do things like pick up a pencil or walk out the door, but it does not control the bodily functions nor a host of other subtle yet powerful functions, such as the images in your mind. The subconscious is an extremely powerful a vehicle within us which can easily control the body's weight.

Extremely Complex Mental Operations, Freud Decided, Were Possible in the Dream State Without the Cooperation of the Conscious Mind

Freud's dream research led him to the conclusion that "thought impulses continued into sleep." He divided them into five groups, which were all incomplete thought processes left over from the day's events.[1]

These were unsolved problems, suppressed thoughts, interrupted thoughts, unsettled impressions, and most importantly to us in the thinking thin process, thoughts which were begun during the day and then continued by the subconscious during sleep.

Dr. Robert D. Updegraff, in his article, "The Conscious Use of the Subconscious Mind,"[2] discusses the importance of relaxing while feeding images to or tapping the inner wisdom of the subconscious. As everyone knows, the most brilliant discoveries have often occurred to inventors who were admittedly *not* working at the time.

Updegraff goes further, to our benefit, by telling us we can consciously make the subconscious mind work for us by giving it a definite, focused assignment and then forgetting it! It's best if you do this right before some relaxing activity or sleep. The subconscious mind will then most likely finish the job.

---

[1]   *Learn While You Sleep*, David Autis, Libra Books, 1964.

[2]   *Readers'Digest*, March, 1960.

According to experts on the subconscious such as Freud, Hollander, and Jung, a wonderful phenomenon occurs when new information is fed into the subconscious image banks. It filters the information back to the conscious mind as needed. Which means, once you have retrained your subconscious mind to "think thin" it will continue to perpetuate those thought patterns even when challenged by other people, the media, the mirror, or old thought forms.

What you eat, do, or say will be driven by new images in the subconscious. You'll learn how to feed these new images into the subconscious through the exercises in chapter five. The subconscious mind is like a giant memory bank. It remembers everything you thought, said, read, saw, were told, and studied today. Feeding it your own conscious choice of thoughts and images will counterbalance any undesirable ones that got stuck there unconsciously.

The Subconscious Mind Will Seek Out Your Goal Against All Odds

According to Van Fleet, in his book, *Hidden Power: How to Unleash the Power of Your Subconscious Mind*,[3] the subconscious mind is a "goal-seeking mechanism." There is no need to be concerned about how your subconscious will work on your desired outcome, because the means will be taken care of simply by focusing on the goal.

---

[3] Fleet, Van, *Hidden Power: How to Unleash the Power of Your Subconscious Mind*, Parker Publishing, 1987.

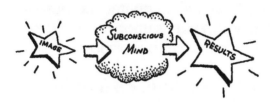

I have found this to be true in thinking thin or any other endeavor I gave to the subconscious to handle! It almost seems too simple, too good to be true, but it does work.

Something You Can Do Now:

Remember a time when you have wanted to do something but did not know how it would be possible? Did a possibly unexpected solution arise as soon as you let go of it? Write the situation and solution here or in your journal:

_____

The subconscious mind is not capable of making value judgmentsof discerning which images you want to manifest and which would be better left dormant. It works like a computer and will fulfill your requests whether they are good, legal, beautiful, wise, or just garbage! It is up to your conscious mind to discriminate between legal and illegal, moral or immoral, beautiful or ugly, etc.

In *The Lively Mind*,[4] by Jules Willing, he tells us that the mind is the "ultimate computer" because it constantly enhances itself and expands upon its own capacity. What a powerful tool we have at our disposal!

Put Your Subconscious to Work While You Sleep

One of the best times to put the subconscious to work for you is while you are sleeping. The subconscious mind never stops processing and manifesting images, even when you are asleep. In fact, some of your dreams may reflect your thinking thin process. Willing calls dreams the "universal language" and says you should regard them as "your own form of mental communication with yourself."

Willing (among many other experts in psychology and spirituality) says you can use this "dreaming self" to "expand the range of your mental activity." He also refers to scientists who have "slept on" a problem, only to wake up with complete and whole solutions, sometimes in the form of new inventions.

---

4 *The Lively Mind*, Willing, Jules, Z.W. Morrow, 1982.

Something You Can Do:

When was the last time you "slept on" a question or problem waking up with a clear idea of what to do about it, or simply a better understanding of it? Write your experience here or in your journal:

_____

Willing recommends "mulling over the problem as you are falling asleep. Some people find it useful to 'resolve ' to solve it while they are sleeping, to 'command' their minds to deal with it." Chapters five and seven show you how to use the dream state in resolving issues relating to weight.

Understanding the Language of the Subconscious is Vital

It makes sense that if you want to speak with someone from a different country, you must know at least some of their language. Luckily, the language of the subconscious mind is something we all use every day. It is just a matter of being aware of how we use it, and discriminating for positive results in our lives.

If we speak to the subconscious mind in its own language, which is a series of vivid images, it will not only produce the image, but it will compel us to manifest the image in some way in our outer lives. It is absolutely uncanny to see this work. You may want to try some of your own simple experiments with this, just to prove to yourself that this really does work.

Try this experiment right now. There is a children's game that says, "Don't think of a hippopotamus." What is the very first thing that came to mind? Was it the words? Of course not, it was the image of the hippopotamus, perhaps followed by the words and the conscious awareness of what the words meant.

Think how this applies to weight loss. What if someone said (I'm sure you have heard *someone* say this before), "I feel so fat!" or "I'm sure I am gaining weight." This person has just given their subconscious mind a command to gain weight.

By reversing the phrasing, one reverses the image, resulting in a more desirable outcome. I would suggest a key phrase as part of the daily diet of thoughts such as, *"I feel so thin!"*, or if that is too unbelievable just yet, *"I feel a bit thinner today."* Or simply repeat the word "thin" to yourself.

The Subconscious Does Not Hear Negatives

If someone were to say, "I'm not going to gain any more weight." The subconscious mind would hear, "I'm going to gain more weight." This is so important to remember, that I am mentioning it several times.

The subconscious works in images. Whatever image you create with your words is exactly what your subconscious will interpret as a command. It's much like throwing a picture down a well to the genie at the bottom of the well who makes it come true in the exact image you have drawn.

It's almost scary to think of the pictures we throw at ourselves on a regular basis. Can you think of anyone you are as critical of as yourself? I can't think of anyone of whom I am as critical. The people I see around me who seem to be so critical of others are probably harder on themselves than anyone, and when I have spoken with them heart to heart, it is always the case.

How You Talk to Yourself is the Image You Are Creating of Yourself

A little known secret of success, as any truly successful athlete, business-person, artist, musician, or actor will tell you, is their own creative imagination and the way they talk to themselves. They may not use the same words I do, of course, but they may say something like, "I never even thought about failing," "I always knew I would win," or "I just saw myself succeeding— I wouldn't accept anything less."

Can you imagine one of these people getting really down on themselves very often, saying things like "I'm really overweight," "I'll never make it," or "No one can love me when I look like this."

Here are a few qualities of winners to study:

Winners are guided by their own standards and beliefs, not other's. What do you want to look like, feel like, be like?

Winners assume command because they are used to accepting full responsibility for themselves. Who do you want to be in control of your body?

Winners are happy, cheerful people with a positive outlook on life. Why not be happy now about the success you are surely going to attain?

Read some success stories on your own to find out more about what winners have in common. Consider reading one story a month about someone who overcame great odds or succeeded in sports or business. You will begin to see the common attitude of quiet determination that runs through each story. People who succeed seem to have this rope they hang on to that says "I'm a winner, I will succeed and I know I am already there." When they get to the end of their rope in any particular situation, they tie a knot and hang on tight!

Like most people, I can be very hard on myself. I remind the subconscious that I don't have to be perfect. Giving myself permission to be less than perfect frees me up to learn more about life. I watch children. The really little ones who are just learning to walk feel good about themselves and their goal no matter how many times they fall.

They hardly ever cry from disappointment until someone starts telling them they're making mistakes! Until that point, they are simply learning from the misstep to step differently. No judgment. It's like a game. Have you ever played hopscotch? When you miss it's kind of fun and makes the game a much more interesting challenge than when you do it perfect every time. Maybe this is the secret appeal of solitaire.

Who Controls the Subconscious Mind?

Your higher self, the real you, Soul, can be in control of the subconscious mind. Thinking thin works best when you see yourself as much more than just your mind or body. You are a divine spiritual being! Here is an exercise to put you in touch with this part of yourself.

Something You Can Do Now:

Imagine you are being handed a bouquet of your favorite flowers. You can feel the crisp coolness of the stems in their green paper wrapper. You smell the wonderful familiar fragrance of the petals. You feel elated to receive them and thank the giver, asking what they are for. He or she says they are in honor of your success in achieving your goal of becoming slimmer and more beautiful, or however you wanted to become.

You were just imagining a scene that you could not view with your physical eyes because they were looking at words on a page. And it wasn't just the mind, because you can definitely stand apart from your thoughts and observe them too. No, there's a part of you that is always watching your thoughts, emotions and physical surrounding with serene detachment. That's not the subconscious, but divine Soul, the true you in your highest self.

As Soul, you are always observing and bringing into reality whatever you have your attention focused on. Free choice is our birthright. Some things take longer than others to bring into being due to our past images and the lessons Soul needed to learn along the way to the goal. Nonetheless, we *will* bring anything we want into being eventually with persistent attention via focused, feeling imagination.

Getting all of the above parts of ourselves to work in harmony as one unit can accomplish miracles. James T. Mangan discovered this principle which he explains in his book, *The Secret of Perfect Living.*[5] He listened to his higher self and found out that if he repeated the word "together" over and over again, his higher self, mind, and subconscious mind would work together for his best interest.

Out of this simple repetition (not thinking at all of what the word meant, just repeating it), he came up with many other words that were health and life-changing. He called them "switches." In a way, that is what your new images do. They "switch" you from one mode to another, from one way of being to another.

Thinking Thin Continues to Work Without Diets

Thinking thin helps to change the image you have of yourself over time, which perpetuates your success. This has occurred in my case and has kept me slim for over ten years. The more I think I am thin, the more I eat, walk, talk, and act like a thin person. The more I act like a thin person, the more people perceive me as thin. And the more I continue to act and automatically eat thin, the easier it is to maintain a comfortable, desirable weight.

---

[5] *The Secret of Perfect Living*, Magnan, James T., Prentis-Hall, 1963.

Thinking thin is a self-perpetuating phenomenon which continues to amaze me. I still find myself changing eating patterns from long ago when I thought I would not have enough to eat, or when I thought I could not eat certain foods.

I now find myself buying a favorite ice cream and leaving it in the freezer for days because I don't have time or inclination to eat it! Does that sound like someone who used to be overweight? I still love to eat good food and I still like to cook very much. I might bake a lemon meringue pie and eat it for breakfast, lunch and dinner, but never gain a pound! I may not eat desert for a day or two after, so it always balances itself. But the point is, I'm not forcing the issue through willpower. Thinking thin helps me be thin naturally.

For the most part, I eat very healthily simply because I imagine myself as a very healthy person. This drives the subconscious to desire foods that are good for me. When I do bake a lemon meringue pie, it is a wholesome one with a whole grain crust and honey for sweetener, and could be considered a very good meal.

Seeing Other People in a Positive Light Helps You See Yourself That Way Too

An essential part of thinking thin for me has been to view other people as Soul, and not as their bodily image. I also look for the beauty that is there, no matter in how small a way. Perhaps it is the eyes, the person's manner, way of speaking or calm beingness.

This serves several surprisingly practical purposes. First of all, it focuses my attention on something other than "fat or thin," no matter who it is.

Secondly, it requires that I make no judgments, about myself or about others. If I were to judge someone else harshly, it would only be an extension of being hard on myself (it is very subtle, but I watch myself do this.) Third, it induces feelings of kindness and the habit of granting freedom. If I allow others to be who they are and have the experience they need for themselves, it allows me room to do the same in my own state of consciousness.

It is not that I do not see the weight of the person, and feel something about it. I simply try to shift my attention to a higher perspective, seeing the inner beauty that person has, in whatever part of them I can find it. When I do have a judgment or opinion about someone else's body weight or shape, it just reminds me of how fearful I have been about looking very overweight. This is partly due to all of the information we are constantly fed about how terrible it is to be heavy in this society. Being large is simply an informational experience for Soul. I tell myself in those moments that it is an experience for those who have chosen it consciously or unconsciously, but it need not be my experience. I have chosen to consciously change that part of my life and am constantly vigilant to hold healthy, slim thoughts.

Even When I "Bloat Up," I Have Learned to Maintain Thin Images

We all go up and down a few pounds in weight. I have had to repeatedly tell myself when I have gained water weight for one reason or another that it is only temporary. I will return to my thin self in a day or two.

This seems to satisfy my subconscious, as long as I do not put fearful thoughts and images in about how *"I must be gaining weight back!"* If I find myself saying things like that, I simply remember the subconscious mind works in images. This sobers me up very quickly to the fact that I must constantly watch the pictures I am feeding myself.

Following the above maintenance of the mental machinery allows me to manage my weight without dieting and has done so for half of my adult life.

You Can Do it Too, Just Like These Other People

One woman who owned a beauty salon saw a flyer for one of my thinking thin workshops. She liked the idea of thinking thin, so without reading or hearing anything more, she decided to develop the process on her own, just as I had.

When I met her, she had been using positive imaging methods for several years. Not only did she have a gorgeous figure, she had decided she didn't like exercising and would try toning her muscles with her mind. It worked! Somehow the images sent to the subconscious mind induced it to keep her muscles busy enough to be toned.

Another woman I met who I'll call Beth discovered these very effective weight reduction principles almost by accident. She had been trying to lose weight, but nothing worked. One night she went to a Leon Russell concert and he was performing a song about his girlfriend named Emily. Emily was on stage with him and was, according to Beth, twice as big as Beth was at the time, even though Beth was pretty hefty herself !

Beth said to me, "She was obviously the woman he loved, and I thought, Well, look at her, she's really big and fat and he's written how beautiful she is, calling her his sweet Emily. He immortalizes her. Then I thought, I can do that too. It doesn't matter what I look like. I can have people love me for what I am.

"I just went home and started melting away. I stopped dieting and went down three pants sizes, eating ice cream sundaes! That was practically all I ate all summer. I suddenly saw the connection. I was feeling good about myself, thinking and feeling like a thin person. I lost a pound every day I ate one of those sundaes. I knew I was losing weight without dieting, and I knew I could eat whatever I wanted and that I wasn't starving to death. I was treating myself. I don't think I ate much else. I loved those sundaes and I loved feeding them to myself. (Now, I am *not* recommending sundaes for lunch every day, because it may not be the healthiest thing, but this person stumbled across a principle that worked for her by accident—that of loving and celebrating herself just the way she was, relaxing and eating whatever she wanted, just as a thin person would.)

Beth continues her story by saying, "I got really excited after a few weeks of losing weight. I'd never before felt satisfied with the way I looked. It was a new sensation.

"As the pounds began to peel away, people started asking me what I was doing to lose weight. I would tell them I was eating an ice cream sundae every day. They'd exclaim, 'Well it can't be that! You're doing something else.' They would try to make me see how I must be dieting.

"My father would argue with me constantly, saying That can't work.' So I would try to find a logical explanation. When I couldn't, I thought, 'It can't work anymore.'

"Then someone else said, 'If you don't stop, you're going to lose too much weight and you are going to melt away.' I got scared because I did not know at that point how to stop losing. But now I do. The letting go and accepting my fatness *was* thinking thin, because I accepted myself as I truly was. A sign I saw during this time expressed what I felt: 'Underneath all this fat is a very thin body!'

Another example of a successful use of thinking thin principles was from a woman I'll call Margaret. She'd read my book and practiced the techniques just five minutes a day. Margaret said she was not a very disciplined person. "The very idea of a diet makes me upset. So doing something without willpower or effort is right up my alley!"

Margaret said she enjoyed the exercises because she could do them easily. She pictured herself the way she wanted to look, and held this key image in her mind for a few minutes each day. "The best thing," she said, "is that it works! It really does work! I was simply amazed at the results I got right away. It has been about two months since I began thinking thin and already I've lost a dozen pounds!

"Now that doesn't seem like much to some people, but to me it means a lot. I didn't have to eat funny; I didn't have to take up jogging or exercise; all I had to do was see myself the way I'd like to be.

"Even my husband commented on how slim I was becoming and he *never* notices things like that. And he rarely hands out compliments, so when he said, 'You're becoming positively skinny, woman!', I nearly fell over!"

Thinking Thin Can Work For Anyone

Thinking thin works simply because the subconscious mind will carry out the orders given it via the imagination. Whatever we think, dream, feel, imagine and focus our attention on will surely come to pass. One of the oldest books in the world, the Bible, says, "As a man thinketh, so does he become." I have no doubt this applies to woman as well!

Dr. Wayne Dyer wrote a book called, *The Sky's the Limit.*[6] In it he talks about the "no-limit" person; one who has the ability to master his or her own health, wealth, or anything else in life that one wants to achieve. It doesn't require special genes or education, but simply a desire to be the best you can be. You must be willing to accept the challenges that go with learning anything new (like changing a flat tire when you have never done it before).

---

[6] *The Sky's The Limit*, Dyer, Wayne, Simon and Shuster, 1980.

He makes a good point in saying, "Why be here anyway?" We have chosen to remain alive and among the living, so why not make it the best we can? I highly recommend his books for an uplift and a "can-do" feeling, as well as proof to yourself and your mind that yet another person has made great life changes against all odds. The main thing your mind needs to be convinced of is that the controls are inside you, not outside.

Even if everything outside of you tells you that you look a certain way, you *always* have the option to disagree. You have the power and the right to imagine yourself the way you want to be. In doing so, Soul creates change. Your divine gift is imagination, and you have the free will to use it as you choose. What do you choose?

There is No Need to Concern Yourself With the "How"

Remember, the subconscious mind does not question the images you feed it. It acts almost like a genie in a bottle. If you know the magic words, you can start it working in your conscious favor. It just takes gentle, persistent "commanding" in the form of a focused image.

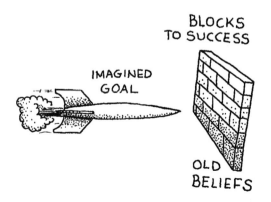

Life eventually brings you everything you need to fulfill this image, no matter what seems to be in the way or how impossible the end result may seem. The subconscious mind has more ability to solve problems and be creative than our conscious minds can conceive. So don't even try to figure out how it is going to work, just experiment with it in a relaxed way—and watch apparent miracles occur!

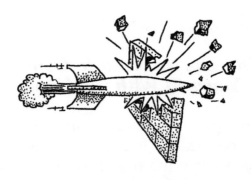

Are there lots of blocks in the way of your goal, or seeming challenges to ever accomplishing it? Remember the subconscious mind is a goal-seeking mechanism, sort of like a heat-seeking missile.

Something You Can Do Now:

Is there any doubt still left in your mind still that you
may not be able to achieve your goal for one reason or
another? Try this exercise. Write all the obstacles that
stand between you and your goal:

_____

Now close your eyes and focus on the key image that
embodies your goal. Imagine that this key image fires up
a subconscious missile that blasts right through each obstacle as it moves swiftly toward your goal. Visualize your
new shape and say aloud, "I am so happy that I actually
did this. I made it to my goal, even though I had some
challenges to meet."

When you can imagine from the end of your goal, it
will build your belief that it is achievable. And when you
believe you can be everything you want to be, you have
already set the reality in motion!

The following chapter will give you all the practical
tools you need to fulfill your dreams of a new you. It is
now up to you to use them, as only you can decide how
fast you want to go on the road to your new reality.

Chapter 5

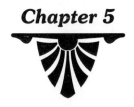

How to Think Thin

"The first step to better times is to imagine them."
— fortune cookie

How Do You Know What You Want to Look Like

In order to begin the process of thinking thin, it may be important to understand just how inundated we are with false images. As Sondra Ray mentions in the prologue of her book, *The Only Diet There Is*,[1] the fashion industry began years ago hiring models who were very thin because the shapelier, more voluptuous figures overshadowed the designer's clothes. The female standard of today is now the skinny image that was originally chosen due to its lack of appeal!

The media today continues to promote this unnaturally thin image with diet soda commercials that employ teenage girls to represent all women. The implication, of

---

[1] *The Only Diet There Is*, Ray, Sondra, Celestial Arts, 1981.

course, is that if you don't look like this nymph at age 38, you should be drinking the diet soda!

How do men feel about very thin women? I heard two men talking recently who had very thin models for mates. The first man said he felt as though his girlfriend was starving herself to death. When he saw her without clothes on, he almost wanted to cry. The other man said he felt like he was getting in bed with a bicycle! Take your own poll and find out what the opposite sex really likes. You may be pleasantly surprised to find that most men like a few curves.

The image you want to create for yourself can be whatever you choose. This could include being heavier, the same weight but with the flesh distributed differently, more feminine, stronger, healthier, more youthful, or simply happier with who you are right now.

I Had to Accept Myself and My Body Before I Could Change It

Before I was able to think myself thin, I learned to see my body as beautiful just the way it was. The more I saw the beauty in it, the more others would see it and comment on it. I accepted the compliments as graciously as I could, imagining they were true.

How did I accept my body? I was fortunate to do some modeling for a group of professional artists when I was in college. At the time I was definitely overweight. The artists were sick of "twiggy-figure" models, as they put it. They told me they were ecstatic to have a model with "rubenesque curves" to give them something interesting to draw! That bolstered my waning self-confidence over the years.

I still carry their kind words with me so I can feel good about my body, no matter what "imperfections" exist. *Absolutely no one* has a Barbie-doll or Ken-doll body. Everyone has something that they wish they could change, no matter how perfect they may look to you. The only way out is to appreciate the beauty in those imperfections and see the character and personality they bring to your life. Our bodies are miraculous vehicles for interesting life experiences and if we appreciate and love them, they will take us much further.

Something You Can Do:

Try this appreciation exercise right now, and see how good you feel afterwards:

Start with your feet, working your way up to the very top of your head and appreciate every muscle, organ and gland you can possibly think of, telling each one how much you love it. Thank each cell and part for everything it has done for you over the years, smiling all the while.

Try to do this on a regular basis, when you are showering, or sitting somewhere quietly. Not only will you love your body more, but it will be healthier as well.

Recrafting My Own Image Came After Self-Acceptance

After I felt better about who I was and accepted the way my body looked, I could start creating what I wanted for my body from a position of loving it. Good Health was my top priority. No matter what I weighed, I wanted to be healthy and energetic.

From my modeling experience, I felt that this country had put way too much emphasis on females resembling toothpicks. This is not only unappealing to most men (and in fact many men are very attracted to larger women), but has caused a great deal of illness in the form of anorexia and bulimia.

No other country in the world has such a neurotic idea about female beauty. The Italians would love us all and in the Hawaiian culture, more fat is more "mana", or spirit. Down through history, large men and women were often considered to be more powerful and more beautiful. How you wish to look should be your own personal choice.

I wanted to create an image for myself that was healthy and attractive according to my standards, not anyone else's. I knew I could love and accept myself no matter how I looked, because I was *not* a body, I was a divine Soul. And as Soul, I could be of service and a vehicle of love no matter what my size.

The process of thinking thin for me began with mental discipline. I decided to think of myself only in thin terms. I threw out my scales, refusing to let them rule me, and began to "catch the feeling" of how it would be to experience a firm, strong, lean, yet feminine body. The feeling was one of being in top-notch condition, energetic, fit and ready for anything!

I faced my fear of food by eating whatever I wanted. I found myself eating differently after a while. I listened to my body first, eating what I felt drawn to. Later, as I lost my love-hate relationship with food, I listened more to my higher self and found out what I needed for optimum health. Now I just eat what I want, knowing that my higher self, my subconscious, and my body are much more in harmony with each other as I choose my foods. It turns out I prefer lots of fresh vegetables, whole grains, and pretty healthy fare now, but I still love *real* butter and eat it!.

Without any forced feeling of will-power or self-discipline, I found myself joining a health club. It was something I *wanted* to do because it seemed fun. As it turned out, the health club was a woman's health club, and many of the women there were interested in body building. I easily slipped into working out with weights. It just seemed natural, enjoyable, and an exhilarating challenge to see how much weight I could lift, press, or push.

As I watched my body change, it amazed me to see how it was becoming just what I had imagined; strong and lean, yet still softly feminine. Later, there were still other things I felt like changing about it, which I proceeded to focus on and alter. In Chapter 10, Beyond Thinking Thin, I'll tell you more about those areas.

Choosing Your Ideal Image

The image I put my attention on was what I became. And believe me, if I can do it, you can too! Since the imagination works very specifically according to the images fed it, it's crucial to choose the image that *you* want to create, not what someone else may want. How would you feel most comfortable with yourself? We know some things about our bodies aren't going to change, at least not without major surgery or Miss Clairol! But other characteristics are within our control.

Here are some areas of possible change you may want to consider before doing the following brief exercise. Feel free to include any areas you want to focus on that aren't listed too:

Health
Energy
Body Mass
Flexibility
Strength
Metabolism
Coordination
Athletic Ability
Attractiveness
Silhouette
General Appearance

Something You Can Do Now:

Write here or in you journal how you would describe the ideal you, physically:

_____

There Are Basic Rules Essential to Thinking Thin

Before applying the techniques listed below, please be aware that the following principles will make a monumental difference as to whether or not the techniques work. Please take these guidelines to heart if you want to be successful. They have been proven over the centuries to bring success in your endeavor.

1. Share this idea with *only* those you trust to support you in it fully, who have your best interests in mind and seem to be positive, forward-thinking individuals. The reason for this is that some people may *unconsciously* sabotage your ideas due to their own inadequate self-image. It's enough of a challenge to meet our *own feelings* of negativity and conquer them, let alone someone else's! In fact, you may want to tell no one until you have proven to yourself that thinking thin works.

2. When creating phrases to repeat to yourself, leave out all negatives such as "no, never, won't, shouldn't, none, don't, etc. Whenever thinking of a phrase with one of these words in it, say to yourself, *"cancel"* or *"erase"* and replace it immediately with a positive reversal. For example: Replace *"I am not fat,"* with *"I am thin."* Notice how this changes the mental image. Remember, images are the sole language of the subconscious.

3. Relaxation while doing any kind of life-changing work is vital. The subconscious is much more receptive when we are relaxed and the conscious mind has been calmed. The easiest way to accomplish this, I have found, is to use your focused imagination techniques just before falling asleep, first thing upon awakening, or just after stretching or exercising. As much new research has shown, if the body is relaxed, the mind is relaxed, because the mind and body are really not separate.

The Following Exercises For the Subconscious Are Essential Tools

The simple tools that follow are crucial in determining the results you will have on this program. Just reading them will not even scratch the surface of your subconscious. You must practice at least one of these exercises on a regular, daily basis, and more than once a day is better.

Make them a vital part of your life. One week of practice will not bring results. You must dedicate yourself to these exercises for as long as it takes to "change your mind" about yourself. The time it takes to do that will be entirely individual.

Always begin with some sort of relaxation exercise. You can use the ICS ("Instant Calming Sequence"), one of your own, or one of those given here. Whatever you do, choose one relaxation technique and stick to it until you feel you need a change, then try another.

Relaxation Exercise #1

Your Own Key Relaxation Image May Work Best For You

Write here or in your journal the most relaxing experience you have ever had:

_____

Just before you begin your exercise for the day, think of this experience to form a "key relaxation image."

Relaxation Exercise #2

Instant Calming Sequence

For an "instant calm" when you are in "panic mode" and want to relax, use this special technique shared by Dr. Robert Cooper. Dr. Cooper explains the technique in detail in his book, *Health and Fitness Excellence.*[2] It is so effective that it can actually calm people who are in a total panic. For your purposes, it can be used whenever you want to practice your exercises during the day.

In order to get a full understanding of this method, called ICS, or Instant Calming Sequence, you may want to read Dr. Cooper's book. I will give you a brief sketch here. It is in five steps and can be done in about five seconds with practice. Practice it when you're calm, so it will be second nature when you need it.

1. Remember to breathe: Breathe smoothly, deeply, and evenly without interruption.

2. Make a Positive Face: Even the slightest smile may reset the nervous system. This technique has been recommended for years in the martial arts. You can also smile inwardly.

3. Balance Your Posture: Imagine a thread gently lifting your whole spinal column upward from the top of your head. Become light and loose, chest open and upward, shoulders down, stomach relaxed, jaw loose.

---

[2] *Health and Fitness Excellence*, Cooper, Robert, Houghton mifflin, 1989.

4. Relax: Do a "tension check scan" through your entire body, and as you do, "Flash a mental 'wave of relaxation' through your body, as if you're standing under a waterfall that sweeps away all unnecessary tension."

5. Control the Mind: Accept whatever situation you're in and command your mind to quickly seek solutions that will work. (In thinking thin, remember your key image—the new you that you are creating).

Practice the above techniques daily.

Relaxation Exercise #3

Clouds Can Be Very Relaxing Images

Think of the most relaxing music you know. Begin to breath gently, yet deeply, telling yourself to relax. As soon as you breathe out, feel each part of your body letting go of any tension. Beginning with your feet, move up through your legs, hips, torso, arms, chest, neck and head.

See clouds of feathery white floating through skies of blue. Now imagine they are floating all through your body. See yourself in a beautiful setting, wherever you most like to go to "get away from it all."

You are now in touch with the "real you," and can be most effective in focusing your imagination on what you really want.

Believe it or not, just by taking the time to relax and imagine for a few moments a day, you will begin to see subtle changes taking place in your life.

Relaxation Exercise #4

Zen Monks Have Relaxation Methods We Are Just Beginning To Use

Whenever you need to clear your mind, gaze gently at a blank wall for a few moments. If you find your eyes wanting to close, let them, and look at the blank screen of the mind.

To extend this exercise in to a deeper relaxation, sing or repeat phrases that are dear to you from your spiritual life. Many religions have a song, prayer, mantra or something using sound to relax and focus the inner being. I have found that these sounds are very healing, focusing, and relaxing for me. They allow the subconscious to be open to just about anything you wish to feed it.

If you can't think of one, here is a simple word sung for relaxing, used for thousands of years by various cultures and religions around the world. The world Hallelujah was derived from the word Hu (pronounced like hue), which was even used by the Navajos for their holiest ceremonies. It is an ancient love song to God. When sung in a long drawn out breath (Huuuu...) it will bring you a feeling of peace, contentment, relaxation, and divine love. No matter what religion you are or aren't, it fits in. It is the common thread that weaves it's way through all time and all people, and especially all sounds. If you listen for it, you can hear it in the wind, music, and even cars! Everything makes this sound, and it will bring you closer to the highest within you. That's the very *best* place to start any of these exercises.

Think Thin Exercise #1

Setting Your Goal in Writing Will Solidify It

Look at what you wrote about your ideal self-image at the end of Chapter 1, and then in the exercise at the beginning of this chapter under "Choosing Your Ideal Image." Review in your mind what you would like your body to look and feel like. Combine the most important features of your ideal body image here or in your journal, using the two written descriptions and what your imagination has just suggested:

Writing down your goal as vividly and completely as possible is vital to success. I write down goals for everything I want to accomplish. I am careful what I write, for I know I will surely attain it!

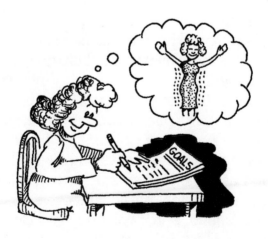

For example, if I want to attend a play, I will write it in my daily appointment book, just as if I am making an appointment with myself. And sure enough, I often find myself in a theater before the week is out.

I record all kinds of goals this way. If I remember to do it, I even write down what new clothes I would like to have by a certain date, or what new lessons I would like to have learned. Be as creative as you wish.

Think Thin Exercise #2

Knowing How Your Goal Can Be of Service Helps You Accept It

How is the new you going to be of greater service to God, your family, loved ones, and yourself? Sometimes people feel that they are not quite worthy of the time and attention necessary to accomplish a purpose that seems like it is "just for them" alone. Here is your opportunity to see how creating a new image of yourself will benefit everyone around you— and all life.

One woman at my workshop felt guilty about taking the time to focus so much on herself. Deeply religious, she did not think it was the most Christian thing to do. But even as she voiced her objections, she realized she had *already* been focusing too much attention on herself in a negative way with regard to her weight. By focusing positive attention on herself, she could change the situation. This would eventually remove the need to pay so much attention to her weight— and free up her energy to love life and God more.

Do this exercise to find out how your self-change work will be of service: First, use the "cloud" relaxation exercise above to get in touch with the real you, Soul.

Now ask that inner self what your goal should be for the healthiest, most optimum shape this lifetime. How will that new image be of greatest service to you and to all those around you?

Rewrite your new image from this viewpoint. Has it changed any? If this seems like you're rewriting the same thing, you are! Repetition of new ideas is the only way to make a dent in the subconscious when it has been pelted with the old ideas for what seems like centuries! There are more writing exercises here which will help you see how much control you really do have over the way you look.

Think Thin Exercise #3

Your Key Image Will Unlock the Door to the Future

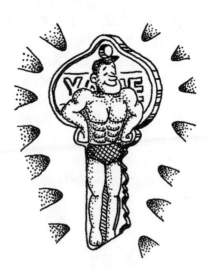

For many of the exercises in this chapter, and in most basic exercises for the subconscious, a key image is of utmost importance. It anchors the mind to the ultimate fulfillment of your goal. When too many scattered, different images are presented, the subconscious becomes confused as to what direction to take.

Television commercials know this principle. They repeat the same commercial so many times you begin to sing the jingle in it and start buying the product. They have presented the same key image over and over again to the subconscious. Instead of the subconscious genie saying, *"Your wish is my command"*, it pronounces, *"Your image is my command."*

Children are very open to subconscious reprogramming. An overweight eleven-year-old girl attended one of my workshops and decided to see herself as her Skipper doll (Barbie's younger sister). She meditated on this image a lot during the day.

Two weeks later, she had lost two dress sizes and 20 pounds! She says her key image has become an imaginary habit. I asked her if she had any advice for people trying to think thin. She said, "Yes. If you don't have the greatest imagination, build it up!"

Now we're ready to write our *key* images. It must be just one scene or picture you can instantly focus upon at any time. Choose the image carefully. What are you wearing? How do you feel? Use all of your senses. If you are by the beach, smell the ocean breeze, hear the waves, and feel the sun on your body. Taste the salt air and look at the sparkling sand. Now write a complete description of your key image, including all of your senses. Put your-self inside the picture, inside the new body, on the beach.

Find a recipe card or any small slip of paper on to which you can copy this key image. On the very top of the card, write in big letters, *relax*. Using your "key relax-ation image" developed earlier in this chapter, or the Zen Zazen method of clearing the mind (gaze at a blank wall), read what you have written often during the day. The *best* times are upon arising and just before sleeping (the subconscious is more open). Also, cue your mind to some key times during the day when you will remember to read your image card. This can be during a break at work, just before or after lunch, every time you get coffee, or when your watch alarm goes off every hour.

Make daily, firm appointments with yourself. Do any-thing it takes to review this key image several times a day. If you can only manage to do the exercise before going to bed and/or upon arising, that is great. As long as you choose consistent times and are persistent, *you will tri-umph*.

When you look at your card, read it in a cheerful and relaxed manner, using all of your senses to fully imagine yourself in key image scene. Add the excitement, con-tentment, or other feeling element you imagine you'll have when you reach that goal. Remember to *put your-self in it*, as if it is true and happening *right now*. Smell it, taste it, touch it, feel it, sense it, hear it, and see what is around you.

Here lies the true secret to success. If you do no other exercise in this book— but do this one faithfully— results are inevitable.

Think Thin Exercise #4

This Basic Exercise is an Extension of the Key Image Exercise

This exercise will take you to the next level of thinking thin by fully experiencing the fulfilled dream. Twice a day, upon awakening and upon going to sleep, set aside 30 seconds. Think of it as the golden minute in your day, something to look forward to because it will make you feel so good.

By thinking of it that way, your mind will feel more motivated to do it. Also, by setting aside specific times to do it, your mind will feel much more comfortable. It likes to work in patterns, or grooves, like a phonograph record. That's why you should always set a regular schedule for anything you want to do. Once you have established that time, your mind will continue to prod you, even when you try to skip your routine. This is why you can't go to bed without brushing your teeth!

The first part of this 30-second exercise is to tell your body that you love and appreciate it just the way it is. Thank it for serving you every day. Tell it you are going to make some changes now that will help you both serve life even better.

The second part of the exercise is to return to your peaceful setting and remember how your new body will be of service.

The third part is to imagine you are in a corner of the ceiling of your room, looking down at your new body. See it exactly the way you would like it to look. Use your key image, if you like, or simply see yourself in bed, looking lean, strong, healthy, or however you want to be. Remember to include the feeling behind the image. That wonderful exhilarating feeling of being in the state of perfect harmony with your physical self.

If it is morning, arise with the feeling of this new body and can carry it with you during the day. If it is nighttime, fall asleep with this image in your mind so your subconscious can work on it overnight. It never sleeps.

This particular exercise works with the principle of assuming the goal fulfilled. All successful people use this principle in one form or another. For example, Jean-Claude Killy, the Olympic Gold Medal winning skier, would see himself skiing a perfect, winning course over and over again.

The first part of the exercise is important too. Sarah found this out when she told herself everyday, *"I love you unconditionally."* She did this while looking deeply into her own eyes in the mirror She told me she tried to mean it with all her heart. The exercise brought her a glow all over and from within, that she called "knowing what God's love has done for me." She would then say to herself, *"You are slim and beautiful!"*

"That was the answer," Sarah declared, "because I am now losing weight without any pills or special diets. Food that is not good for me is now tasteless. I don't even want it.

"When you feel beautiful," she continues, "you want to continue to look beautiful. For me, exercise was like a trial, but now I *want* to exercise. When I do, I keep telling myself, *'I'm beautiful!'*"

Think Thin Exercise #5

Using a Key Phrase to Boost Your Thinking Thin Power

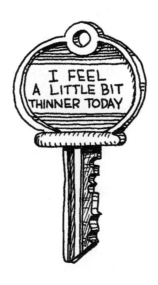

A key phrase is something you say to yourself constantly to create forward-moving images for the subconscious to work on. The phrase can also be used to replace any limiting thoughts or images that might arise during the day. For example, let's say you hear someone talk about dieting or weight and begin to think about your own situation. Immediately take a deep breath, relax your entire body, and begin to repeat your key phrase.

Sometimes just one word works best. That word can be "thin", "slim", "lean" or "light." If you are aiming to become stronger and heavier, as is the case with some people, you might repeat words like "solid", "muscle", "substantial", etc.

Write your key phrase hereor in your journal:

_____

Here are some key phrases from which to choose if you like:

A. *"I am feeling thinner today."*

B. *"I look and feel lighter today."*

C. *"I am going to fit into the next size smaller any minute!"*

D. *"I feel so thin inside, my outside is just about to catch up!"*

Key phrases are very powerful. Most of us have actually gained weight by the unconscious use of key phrases like, *"I feel so fat."* Have you ever noticed that when you repeat those types of phrases with a strong feeling behind them, you see yourself gaining weight?

I used the key phrase, *"I feel a little thinner today."* Every morning before I looked in the mirror I would say to myself, *"I am feeling a little bit thinner today."* Then I would assume that when I looked in the mirror I would *look* thinner too. There were times when I may have actually looked heavier, but I continued to reaffirm my thought and image daily with my key phrase until it "took."

Jean told me she used a key phrase to help her make a major career transition. She was the first woman engineer at a major power company and was valued highly by all, especially the women whom she mentored. When she decided to quit her job and begin her own massage therapy business, she found a way to gain dearly needed support from her friends and associates at work. Her tool was a key phrase.

Every time Jean told someone she was leaving, she would take their hand, and say to the person, "Tell me you will support me in this next step because I am going to quit." She said, "I was affirming that God would support me in what I was about to do, because it wasn't necessarily going to be easy, especially financially.

"But life did support me— I even won a modest amount in a lottery, which showed me I was on the right track. It felt like God and I were playing a game together. When I was in a positive flow, He gently supported me. The only time I felt alone was when I isolated myself from abundance, from love. It's a choice. Be negative or positive.

"When I used to dislike what was happening in my life, I'd say, 'I'm going to bed.' Now I no longer give my outer life or circumstances that kind of control over me. I feel like I'm falling in love with my positive self. I can't do anything now that doesn't honor who I truly am."

Meditation helps Jean in overcoming her weight problem. I asked her advice on changing self-talk. She said, "You have to change self-talk slowly, so you improve bit by bit. You can't feed steak to a baby, so take it easy with yourself when you're just beginning. Work on erasing negatives. You have to hear the negative stuff first, so you see what you're feeding yourself." Listen to your own self-talk for one day a week, say Fridays. Awesome, isn't it? Can you go easier on yourself for just and hour? Try it.

Think Thin Exercise #6

Face Your Fear of Food

You are in control of food, it is not in control of you. Fear is one of the strongest motivators to eat known to man or womankind. Some psychologists who work with overweight people suggest they go out and buy all the foods they fear eating too much of because they love them so much. Familiarity breeds contempt. It is amazing how quickly your fear foods can lose their grandiose appeal.

I don't believe it necessary to go to the extreme of acting this out. Thinking thin allows your to eat whatever you desire. Just tell yourself as you eat that you are thin and that your body needs just exactly what you are eating. You'll find your eating habits changing as the subconscious registers this message! You may even find yourself eating *more*, as is necessary for many of us— it was for me (see suggested reading list in the back of this book, *How to Become Naturally Thin by Eating More*).

If you are going to eat something wild, you might as well enjoy it. I don't know how many times I have eaten a favorite food while ruining my enjoyment with guilt! Does this sound logical or loving? Of course not, but millions of intelligent people do it on a daily basis.

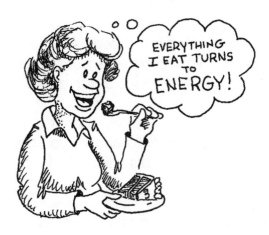

When Thanksgiving comes, most people *expect* to gain weight. Of course, it's not possible to gain that much weight from one meal. But fear and guilt are often the secret fuel that drives us to overeat during the holidays.

Now I just tell myself I am losing weight from all the work my body had to do to digest a big holiday dinner. This keeps me from feeling guilty and beating myself up— which would in turn trigger more overeating out of self-hatred. Now, I simply cannot stuff myself, no matter what time of year it is or how good the food looks. It simply does not satisfy or fulfill me to hurt myself by eating too much food. This includes very high-fat or high-sugar foods. You will find the same to be true as you continue to think thin over the years. But for now, simply enjoy whatever you feel like eating.

Think Thin Exercise #7

Becoming Your Own Script Writer Puts You In Control

The power of writing is just beginning to be discovered by many people. This exercise is not only a very powerful tool to life control, it's a lot of fun as well.

Pretend you are your greatest admirer, someone who could be your life mate, who adores you and thinks you are absolute perfection. This will really be the higher, inner you speaking.

Use your personal journal to write a script of your loved one speaking to the new you: the person you will be after you have accomplished your goal. He/she tells you how wonderful you look, how glowing and healthy and slim (or whatever words you feel responsive to).

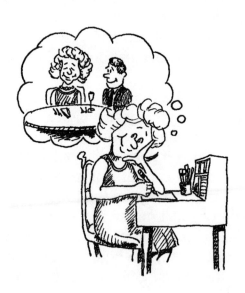

He/she goes on and on about your good qualities, and how becoming your new image is. Go into detail about what you are wearing, and how well it fits and flatters your new figure. Comment on aspects of your body that have changed positively.

Now you are ready to become a script-writer. You will be writing a scene from the play of your day-to-day life. The play is set in your future. I have written the basic scene for you. Rewrite the scene below using the word "I." Add any personal details you choose to better describe the occasion, clothing, people present, comments, and the way you feel. Ready?

You are wearing a dress/suit that is the size you would like to be. It fits perfectly and is the most flattering type of clothing you can think of for your body type. You are walking through a crowd of people, most of whom are your close friends, relatives, or business associates, at a warm gathering of some kind. People begin to recognize you and as you pass by, they stop you and make comments such as, "My, I hardly recognize you! You are so much thinner!" "Congratulations on your new figure!" "How lovely/handsome you look in that new outfit." "What did you do to get so slim?"

As you mingle, eyes turn admiringly, noticing your healthy, glowing shape. You feel wonderful. You have accomplished your goal and feel at peace with yourself. Someone begins to talk about diets, calories, and how much weight they need to lose. You simply listen neutrally or turn your attention to something else. You have absolutely no interest in the conversation because it doesn't apply to you. You are exactly how you want to be and you got there without dieting. The gathering goes on as people continue to shower you with compliments. You accept them with gracious thanks.

As you are writing your "I" script, engage all your senses. Smell the perfume and after-shave, taste the food or beverage, feel the warm touch of your friends, hear their laughter, and the sincerity in their voices as they congratulate you. See the colors of the clothes, makeup, and furniture. Describe all of this in writing, from the first person, or "I," point of view.

A good way to use this exercise: read it to yourself daily before falling asleep or upon awakening. Do it in place of *or* in addition to exercise #4. Remember, the more of these exercises you do, regularly, the faster will be your results.

Think Thin Exercise #8

Recording Your Script on Tape is Very Effective

Make a tape recording of the above script on an audio cassette. You might begin the tape with some soft, relaxing music and your key relaxation image. Tell yourself to relax and listen.

The sound of your own voice is very influential to the subconscious— remember all that self-talk? You can use a different script if you want to, of course. Just keep a specific focus for the script, such as I did with the party.

As you make the tape, replace any "I's" with "You" in the script and remove any negative statements such as "I am not", or "You aren't." Be sure all your sentences create positive, firm, and accurate images to feed the sub-conscious.

Listen to your thin tape before falling asleep, while you're driving, or anytime you feel relaxed. The subconscious will be most receptive as you fall asleep. If you are awake, use your imagination to smell, see, feel, and hear the scene as much as possible. Close your eyes (not while driving!) and put yourself right there in the scene.

This exercise has worked to make my dreams come true, whatever they have been. I listen to my own voice telling me what I already have and fall asleep to it. It is miraculous. I have achieved higher levels of relationships, income, health and well-being as well as inner calm from using a simple tape recorder to send images to my sub-conscious while falling asleep.

I use my own voice because I know exactly what I am saying to myself, in the way I want to say it, using my own specific goals. You can buy a subliminal tape for weight loss, but it will say things from someone else's point of view. I prefer to consciously choose my own images and put in the effort to change my subconscious myself. People also tell me they stop getting any benefit from subliminal tapes as soon as they stop using them. This method will keep working because the "source" is *you!*

There are some wonderful non-subliminal (you hear the words) audio tapes I do recommend by Emmett E. Miller, M.D. They teach deep relaxation. He also has an audible-script cassette called "Imagine Yourself Slim" which may be helpful to those without time or desire to make their own.

Think Thin Exercise #9

Find a Picture of Yourself or Someone else Looking Slim

Marion told me, "I found a picture of a lovely girl with a very beautiful figure and put a picture of my head on it. I put it up at work where I could see it constantly. The visualization is so strong inside that every time I want to indulge I see that figure. I dream it, I am it. That's what keeps me going."

I did something similar by digging up an old high school picture. I look so slim and relaxed in my T-shirt and shorts. I put it on my refrigerator— not to deter myself from eating, but to remind myself that I was thin, no matter what I ate. Of course the change in subconscious imagery to this thin image shifted my metabolism and made subtle changes in my eating and exercise habits.

This exercise won't take up any time in your day. Once you have found a picture of yourself or someone else whose body you really admire (with your head pasted on it), place it where you will see it often; in your wallet, on your mirror, in your car, or anywhere you can think of. Use several pictures for even faster progress.

Think Thin Exercise #10

Listening to Your Higher Self Will Move You in the Right Direction

Many self-help books today recommend that you listen to your body. This is all well and good when you have been used to doing so. But most of us with weight management problems have gotten some very confusing messages from our bodies. Until we can get clear of the turmoil created by our minds, the media, our peers, and our fears, we must look to the still, small voice within. It can guide us to what is best.

Donald was on his way home from work with a craving for Chinese food. He was trying to watch his weight. The particular food he wanted was greasy and not necessarily the healthiest. Should he listen to his body? He knew how to tune into his higher self, and so he did. This innermost self gave him an image of going home to exercise, take a refreshing shower, and then sit down to a light, nourishing meal of brown rice and vegetables. That image felt better to him from his higher viewpoint. He decided to go with what his higher self was telling him through this expanded image. He said the exercise and meal at home was very satisfying. It was rewarding to know he had followed his inner, healthy nudges instead of following old patterns of self-indulgence.

Here is a simple exercise you can use to "tune in" to *your* higher self so it can guide you. Use it until your body is attuned with it automatically (you will know when that time comes).

See a bright, shining star inside you. It grows and expands until it's rays reach out from within you to all of your surroundings. You feel the warmth of the star's silvery-blue glow throughout your body. You *are* this star. What images does this light-being offer?

Doing this exercise right before any of the other exercises will help you make an easier transition to the new you. It speeds up your progress because you are operating from the highest, most expanded viewpoint of all, that of divine Soul.

You can also try it any time you are about to choose something to eat. This may work particularly well for those plagued by eating disorders or food fears.

Think Thin Exercise #11

Dreams Can Change Your Life With Control of Their Imagery

Sherry decided to try this dream technique for "changing her mind" with regard to body image. She started asking for "thin dreams". The first dream she had was of herself when she was a little girl of three years. In the dream she saw a familiar scene. She was swinging on a doorknob, just as she used to do.

When Sherry woke up she thought, *"What a beautiful memory, but what does it have to do with being thin?"* Then she realized how light she had felt in the dream. The whole idea of the dream was to reawaken that feeling of lightness so she could incorporate it into her key image.

The second dream Sherry had was of a sleek, white sport scar. It kept going faster and faster, getting thinner and thinner. The dream was telling her that she would get thinner and also have more energy!

Dreams are invaluable for 1) giving you a positive feeling about what you are doing, 2) gently removing blocks to success, 3) showing you your future image, and 4) revealing what would be best for you to do, eat, or imagine.

Dreams can also be very healing. The next exercise is a simple way to efficiently use that huge block of time we set aside for sleeping. Remember the research mentioned in Chapter 4. The subconscious likes to finish projects the conscious mind has begun, especially while you sleep.

Dream Exercise #1:

Before going to sleep, write any question you may have about controlling your weight in a notebook or in your dream journal (see Chapter 11 for sample dream journal).

Upon awakening— or if you wake in the middle of the night— write down any dream you remember, no matter how silly it may seem. Every dream has some meaning to it. It may seem like a jumble at first, but try this.

Write down any detail you can think of. When you have the whole dream down, tell yourself you know just what it means. Then start brainstorming on paper. Have fun— what does an umbrella mean to you? Protection? Maybe that umbrella your sister was holding over your head means she is an ally in helping you ward off negative self-images. Give her a call next time you're feeling down on yourself.

Another easy way to get the dream message is to write underneath the dream you have logged, "The meaning of this dream is... " and then just let the answer flow out of you.

Dream Exercise #2:

In this exercise you will experience the new you. Simply ask for a dream of your new, slender, healthy, energetic self. Write your request in the dream journal in Chapter 11 or a notebook. Describe how you would like the dream to be. Then fall asleep with that image fresh in your mind. The subconscious will finish your dream for you— and maybe you'll remember it in the morning.

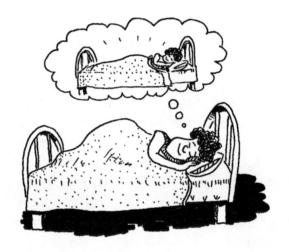

Upon awakening, write down anything you can remember about your dreams, even if it is just *one word*.

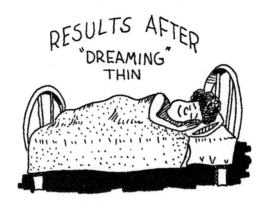

RESULTS AFTER "DREAMING" THIN

Find the meaning in it by using the same method as in dream exercise #1.

There are many good books on dreams and dream interpretation, especially. However, the most important thing to remember is that only you can unlock the meaning of your dreams. Everyone's dream symbols are unique. We each have a different idea of what a word or symbol means according to our individual experience.

Think Thin Exercise #12

Becoming Childlike Opens the Mind to Change

Children have a quality of excitement about new experiences, which to adults may seem mundane. That's because adults think they have experienced them over and over again (even though *every* moment is unique). Kids are willing to believe almost anything and often do— witness the Saturday morning commercials!

Children have a wonderful gift for pretending. This is a valuable skill we can learn from them. Within the spark of imagination is a treasure to be "caught." Have you ever noticed how children become completely absorbed in whatever they are playing? They *become* the image they want to create.

If they're playing pilot, they are really flying that airplane, complete with sound effects, visuals, and leaning sensations. They are above the ground, soaring through the clouds, looking at the tiny world below.

This is the sort of imagination we need if we want to successfully think thin.

Pretending Exercise:

Remember a happy childhood scene. Maybe it's the last day of school in the third grade. The teacher says, "Have a wonderful summer. See you next fall!" You run out of the classroom, so ecstatic at gaining your long-awaited freedom. Or perhaps you linger, tasting the year's memories and saying good-bye to a favorite teacher or friend.

For you it might be a favorite tree house retreat, or playing kick-the-can, or jumping in a pile of leaves. Close your eyes, enter this happy childhood memory, and really relish the feeling of love and freedom. Write it here or in your journal:

_____

Now hold that feeling as you think of yourself as a child now— simply stuck in an adult body! We're about to go on a childlike imaginative journey.

First, imagine yourself as a rock. Pretend you are a big, immovable boulder. How does that feel?

Next, you have been touched by a magician's wand and are turning into a hawk. You fly freely above the earth with the sun on your back, the wind ruffling your feathers as you fly. How does it feel to be so free?

Suddenly you find yourself becoming a feather on the hawk's wing, as it falls away from the wing, gently float-ing to earth, all light and wispy. How does it feel to be so buoyant, weightless and airy?

Whenever you are feeling heavy, immediately begin to pretend. First remember the happy childhood scene— that opens your heart and subconscious to new images. Then think of yourself as a rock-turned-into-a-hawk, and then a feather, lighter than air. You have just eased the mind into a positive state, by using your negative feeling as a springboard into freedom.

Speaking of Children

Here's an exercise for your child who is overweight, but too young to use the "Think Thin" exercises alone, or at all.

When you put your child to bed at night, tell him/her s/he is handsome/ lovely and slim and strong, and that tomorrow s/he will wake up even *more* handsome/ lovely, slimmer and stronger!

Upon awakening, say, "You look so slim and strong. Do you feel slim and strong. The child will probably say "yes." If s/he doesn't, say, "Well, can you *pretend* that you are?" The child will probably say "yes." If not, ask why. Talk about it more or seek professional help.

The Following Ideas Will Help You Reach Your Goal Even Faster

Accept that controlling your weight is a life-long responsibility. You do not have to diet for the rest of your life, nor should you, but you do have to choose a conscious body image to reach and maintain health. The reality is that everything in this world must be reinforced in some way, or it will change. For example, we have to continually wash our bodies, brush our teeth, clean our houses, and keep an income coming in. The same is true of our thought processes. Refuse collects quite easily in the mind, too! Any state you want to perpetuate has to be rewon every day.

Because most of us have been filled with limiting images for so many years, we must also work a little harder as we start thinking thin to counteract old images. There is a trick to doing that. It's like filling a hole with dirt. You always have to pack a little extra on top to allow for settling.

Something You Can Do:

Every time you have a limiting thought or image of yourself, replace it with several positive, new images or thoughts. View your subconscious as a garden. In order to replace weeds with flowers, you must pull up the old, negative thoughts and plant lots of positive seed images every day. The more new images you plant, the stronger and faster your garden will flourish, manifesting a new you.

2. Mock up an ideal image of a personal physician to supervise your thinking thin process. She/he has tailored a special "diet of the mind" for you, as well as an optimum eating and exercise program. Ask the doctor to be your ally when ever you need motivation or advice.

This technique was very effective for me, because I see doctors as positive authority figures. I asked my inner doctor what to eat, how to exercise, and why I should persist. She always helped me out!

3. Keep it simple. Begin with one exercise the first week. Practice it everyday to the best of your ability. Add one exercise per week until you feel you are doing as much as is comfortable. Then just hold to your routine. If you get bored with one exercise, find a different one to replace it with. Stay creative and alert to input from all sides of your life. Your subconscious will attune you to all kinds of subtle assistance. This can come in the form of magazine articles, a story from a friend, a new food at the grocery store, or even a passing comment by a stranger, that will keep you motivated and moving toward your goal.

The more exercises you can do during the day, the faster and more effective this process will be. If your life is very busy, just tackle one simple exercise and practice it faithfully. Do it while showering or brushing your teeth, if necessary!

4. Use as many of your senses as possible when doing the exercises. You don't have to be good at visualization to do these exercises. Some people are more auditory or kinesthetic (hearing or feeling oriented). Use whatever senses you can.

5. Your focused imagination is fueled by feeling. Any strong emotion accompanying your image will cause it to come to fruition much faster. Feel the excitement of accomplishing your goal, the bubbly enthusiasm or happiness you feel being in your new body. Being able to "pretend" or "make believe" as a child would helps. After all, why should kids have all the fun?

Be Creative and Make Up Your Own Exercises Anytime You Want

Use the dream journal in Chapter 11 or your own journal to make up exercises for yourself. Or adapt these twelve key exercises to fit your own personality, spiritual beliefs, and lifestyle. Whatever you feel most comfortable will work best, and should be your priority.

The importance of regularity when doing any exercise for the subconscious— even if it's only one— cannot be stressed enough. The *only* way this book will work is if you *use* it.

In my experience, many people feel it is easier to stick with the exercises when they have a support group of friends or acquaintances who are also thinking thin. See Chapter 8 if you'd like ideas on how to form a Thinking Thin support group.

Most of all, be patient, loving, and kind with yourself. Have fun with the exercises! Feel good about yourself no matter what you eat or do, for you are truly a spark of the divine. You do have the power to change by choosing new images and beliefs.

Your goal will be accomplished if you follow the steps faithfully. Give yourself time. It took years of conditioning to form our beliefs the way they are; it takes a bit of patience to undo them. It took me quite a while! Be persistent in thinking thin, for it will eventually work— and will work quickest of all with constant attention. Good luck!

Chapter 6

What Happens When You Think Thin?

"There are no shortcuts to anyplace worth going."
— Beverly Sills

During the time that I was learning to reshape my body by controlling my thoughts, I began wanting less food or lighter food. But I did not diet. I ate what I wanted and listened as best I could to my innermost self. I felt like joining a health club, so I did. All this was natural. I was simply drawn to what I needed by the subconscious mind's orders to fulfill the image I had given it. I found myself working out with weights. When I remembered the lean but strong body I had envisioned for myself, it all made sense.

This did not happen instantaneously, although it is a very quick process for some people. I did gain a little weight at first, but I was not even aware of it until I looked at pictures of myself months later. I kept holding the image of what I wanted to look like, believing that was how I already looked. Eventually it took hold.

When I started getting close to my desired weight and shape, a friend of mine said to me, "You'd better be careful not to lose too much weight. Your features are angular and will become too sharp looking." It was then that I actually began to *worry* that I might not be able to stop losing weight, that I would get too thin, or worse yet, disappear altogether!

At one point in the process, I did become too thin, so I reversed the process a little and saw myself a little softer for balance. It worked, and I became more of how I am today. I am very happy with the way I feel and look, because I do not expect to look like a mannequin. What really matters is to hold the image *you* want to become. Do not let anyone else provide images for you, unless they are complimentary to your own.

Look For Some Adjustments in Yourself When You Start the Process

Magical things begin to happen. Don't be surprised if you begin to exercise, go for walks, eat differently, cut out sodas, eat smaller, more frequent meals, develop a distaste for rich foods, see a therapist, go to a healing workshop, learn to say no to leftovers, or actually begin to eat *more*! Whatever your particular body needs to do to become the shape you are imagining, it will do— if you let it.

There is a different, individual reason for *every* weight control problem. Each of our minds and bodies are a varied combination of myriad experiences, genes, environment, feelings, personalities, and states of conscious awareness. Thinking Thin cuts through all the complexity with one simple tool: your creative, focused imagination.

As you continue to focus your attention on your key image, you may find yourself doing things you never expected to do, never wanted to do, and never imagined yourself doing. These new patterns are the result of your subconscious, which is cutting through the blocks to weight-control success. You can help the process by acting upon what your higher self is telling you to do.

If you get an inclination to go for walks after dinner, do so! If you keep bypassing the beef at the grocery store, let it be. Your new image is guiding what you do and eat. Even if you get a nudge to do something you have never done before, rest assured that you are on the right track, as you begin to trust the all-knowing part of yourself more and more.

Learning to Listen to Your Higher Self Will Help the Changes Happen

Think of what happens when you turn the channel on a television set. If you see a new program and you like it, you keep watching. Pretty soon you forget you are watching a program. It begins to become very real, until you become a part of it, not just the observer. The only way you know you are really in your living room watching a show is when a commercial comes on and jars you back to your physical location. Thinking Thin is just adjusting your inner awareness and reality to a new channel or frequency of vibration.

Unless you are very aware, listening to your body alone may pull you back to old patterns at first, like the commercials that keep interrupting a good story. Spotting old patterns may be a bit tough too, at first. Listening carefully will assure that the direction in which you move now will be the very best.

Keep practicing exercise ten to "turn the channel" to your higher self, and the program *it* wants to play out. Whenever you find yourself in a quandary about what to eat or do regarding your weight management, listen to that gentle inner voice. The loud voice is usually the one that desires what is not always the best for us, with its alluring charm. The quieter, deeper voice within gives the best advice, and can be trusted as your inner guidance. Some people call it your guardian angel, intuition, following your hunches, the holy spirit, or the voice of God. Whatever you choose to call it, find out for yourself how it works.

When Joanie, the eleven-year-old girl who lost 20 pounds first began thinking thin she listened to her higher self. She had money to get candy bars or sodas if she wanted to. But every day at school, she really felt like getting an apple or banana when she tuned into to the quiet inner voice. By holding on to her key image, and listening to that voice within, she reached her goal. If an eleven year old girl can do it, so can you!

Most People Think They Have to Use Willpower for Weight Control

Joanie acted on her inner guidance by getting the banana or apple instead of the candy bar. She was honoring her highest self and her own health and well-being. The action was not forced, she was quick to note, but just felt natural. When we are really in tune with the inner guidance, things do happen more naturally. You don't have to try, suffer, or force results as one might expect from years of struggle with dieting or exercise.

Consciously notice you are not forcing anything as you use your childlike quality of imagination. You are focusing with a purpose, but from a happy viewpoint of the good things to come. Delightful anticipation fills your consciousness. You feel good about what you eat, what you do, and how you interact with others.

Miriam found herself in the much-too-small size-ten section of a clothing store. She asked herself, What are you doing here? Then she realized, *It's because that's how I think of myself!* "*I'll be back here in a month,*" she promised herself aloud. She has been trimming down steadily. Instead of the pasta with rich sauces, she now asks for salads. That's what works for her. Your body may do fine with rich pasta. The important thing to do is listen and then act, without using willpower.

Taking Action is Essential Once You Feel the Inner Nudge to Do Something

"I feel much more in control of my food," comments Sharon. I was raised on the idea that food equaled prosperity, love and even anger at times. I caught myself wanting to eat when I was upset, and decided to do something healthy for myself instead. People have noticed that I've lost weight. I see it happening slowly."

It's important to look at what issues are tied up with food for you— and then act on those issues. Notice that Sharon saw a pattern of eating whenever she got upset. But she didn't just sit there. Instead, she acted on the nudge from her higher self and consciously substituted another activity or food choice to deal with the issue. It's not using will-power, just making an active choice.

The choice will be much easier and clearer when you stay focused on your key image. The key image will polarize you toward the foods and actions that are in alignment with it. Your job is just to move in this new direction. Don't let old patterns pull you back, simply because you want to stay in the old comfort zone.

Even if you do slide back in to old patterns, you will find you're not as comfortable in them as you were before you began your imaginative reconstruction efforts. After a few weeks of thinking thin I no longer desired the rich deserts I used to find so appealing. They simply do not hold the magnetic attraction they used to. I am just as happy with a light desert or even fruit, if I eat desert at all. I do enjoy sweet tastes, but they seem to continually be taking a healthier, lighter form over the years of thinking thin. It may happen much quicker for some people with vivid imaginations.

The Action You Take May Not Have Anything To Do With Foods

While you have your attention focused on your ideal image, you may find yourself drawn to key information about psychological reasons for weight retention, intriguing exercises, the power of imagination, food allergies, or other issues related to your goal. Someone may recommend a good nutritionist, therapist, diet. Pay attention to these subtle cues— they are your subconscious talking to you!

Keep in mind that there is a unique combination of solutions for your weight management problem because *you* are a unique individual with different chemistry, personality, health, likes and dislikes, and psychological makeup. Approach it like a Sherlock Holmes, open to any clue or thread that leads to a new way of eating, thinking, exercising, or being. The simplicity comes in by just focusing your attention on the goal.

The solution that is right for you will automatically appear. (It may have been there all along, but now you will simply be able to see it more clearly.) The subconscious will be open and seeking answers. Ask it to tip you off when they are staring you in the face! Trust yourself, or at least the ability of your higher self and your subconscious to guide you through this maze.

You May Begin to Like Yourself More Just the Way You Are

Some people report that their shape remains much the same, but they feel differently about it after thinking thin. Even if you are determined to change your body, thinking thin will help you begin to see the beauty in it, as you change you inner image of yourself. It seems paradoxical that you may actually lose interest in being the perfect, svelte physique you have always imagined. Yet when thinking thin, people sometimes wake up to their individuality of shape and size and see it as a work of art, as unique expression of themselves and life.

Everyone will respond differently to this notion. Some people may decide they really do enjoy their bodies, and have simply been fooled by the media and society into thinking it should change. Many women do not realize how thin they are already because they keep believing the media which bombards them with the idea that everyone needs to lose weight. Others may realize they need to change for health reasons and that they truly would feel more comfortable with a different shape.

I found that I got too thin at times and actually had to add some weight in my thoughts. Being skinny didn't feel as good as I thought! Now I feel more comfortable with my body than I ever have before. So do many others who have been thinking thin.

There Are Many Side Benefits to Thinking Thin

Greta says that after attending my thinking thin workshop, she decided she was acceptable the way she was. "I did not need to change physically, but thinking thin has awakened me to the idea that I can control my thoughts and feelings as well as my outer life. Now I'm looking more deeply into myself." Friends tell her she looks much sleeker and happier— probably just from her inner adjustment of attitude!

One of the wonderful benefits of thinking thin, even before your body begins to change, is that other people begin to notice something different about you. They may begin to comment on how great you look, or even how slim you look!

Remember, saying "Thank you" and accepting the compliment will help you to accept your new self too. As you do this, your self-image will improve more and more, perpetuating itself by the compliments you attract with your new "slim and beautiful" attitude.

"I haven't been able to eat sweets like I used to," Greta told me. "I am more attracted to fruits and vegetables." It is obvious that Greta is on her way to a new and healthier body, but more importantly, a whole new self image.

Even People With Eating Disorders Feel More Comfortable With Themselves

People with eating disorders who have used the thinking thin exercises feel much more comfortable with themselves and their bodies. It takes time, but many of them have resolved the deep issues that go along with anorexia or bulimia. Why? Mostly because they have learned to think about themselves in a more positive light. Women tell me they no longer have the need to punish themselves— sometimes a hidden cause behind these illnesses. They use imagination to adjust their self-image to what it really is anyway— slim and feminine.

Attitudes Toward Others Change As Well

Notice how your attitude toward others may change as your attitude toward yourself becomes more loving, accepting, and non-judgmental. You may not feel so judgmental or fearful toward the people around you— even those you used to criticize in photographs, on TV, or in the supermarket.

Your ability to see the unique expression each person is will be enhanced. By paying attention to this ability to give others freedom, you will ultimately find more freedom to think yourself thin. You have unlocked the chains that bound you to the holy grail of the ideal Hollywood image so popular in today's world. Maybe we will be bet-

ter friends to each other when we are all more at peace
with our own images and selves.

Loving acceptance is the key if you have children with
a weight problem. The more they are accepted for exactly who they are, the more likely it is that they will see
themselves more balanced and healthy and thus will become so.

You May No Longer Want to Eat When You Feel Emotionally Upset

The memory is very pale and dim at this point in time,
but I know I used to eat when I was upset, angry, anxious,
lonely, or rejected. Even when I was not in the least bit
hungry, emotionally agitating situations caused me to
head straight for the nearest food. It is very obvious to me
now that I was "stuffing" the emotions down with food. I
did not want to feel whatever I was feeling, so I unconsciously put a lid on the emotions.

These feelings generally arose from my solar plexus,
so I unconsciously made sure they would not go any further by stuffing them back down with food. Many people
do this with food, cigarettes, alcohol, or other drugs. It's a
common solution to a very common problem. The inability to handle emotional stress causes us to want relief.
You may not have an alcohol or drug problem, but you
might be distancing yourself from real emotional issues
with food—especially those you are allergic to.

I know one woman who says that whenever she has to
face a problem at work, she eats croissants in front of the
TV. She's allergic to wheat, so this puts her right to sleep.

It's a way of avoiding the work of consciously facing a problem and tackling it proactively.

We are not taught the basics of how to deal with emotions. Why? Because our parents didn't know how either! It is really very simple, but not necessarily easy. If allowed to occur naturally, emotions arise, are felt and are passed off, like bubbles surfacing on a pond. Most of us are afraid of the pain we will feel if they surface, so we find a way to "put a lid on them" to keep them from surfacing. Food does this very conveniently.

The healthy way to handle emotions, as any therapist will likely tell you, is to go ahead and feel them. This doesn't mean you have to act out of them, but you can let go and experience them to their fullest. You'll find they pass away less painfully. If you need assistance in learning how to experience your emotions without fear, you can get help from a counselor or therapist. More about this will be covered in Chapter 7. Many people who are overweight tell me they are holding back emotionally.

You may find that as you continue to think thin, holding your key image in your attention, you will also allow yourself to feel more. Because you are becoming more relaxed about who you are in life, you may also become more comfortable with feeling however you need to feel and letting the emotions surface. I found a good way to do this without hurting others was to sit down, close my eyes and just feel whatever I was feeling as much as I could. I watched as images and feelings surfaced in a sort of mist that dissipated as it they left my body.

Something You Can Do Now:

If you are feeling the need to eat something because you are emotionally upset, try this experiment:

Tell yourself you can have whatever you want to eat in just a minute. Then sit down in a comfortable chair or lie down somewhere soft and inviting. Breath deeply, exhaling any tension you may feel. Begin to use one of the key relaxation exercises, like singing a favorite hymn or singing Hu and imagining a stream of blue light (very calming) filling the area in your body where you may feel pain or emptiness.

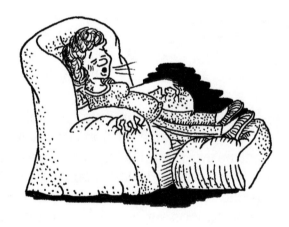

Now simply allow whatever you are feeling to surface. Cry if you want to, or hit a pillow if you feel frustrated. Do allow all emotions to surface and be "passed off". If you feel anger, shoot it toward the center of the earth and let it melt in the molten lava there. If you feel pain, let it dissipate as a mist which becomes clear air as it leaves your body. Use your imagination to bring about whatever healing you can.

A blue light is very effective to shine on any dark spots that still hurt or feel hollow. Let the love of God, spirit, the life force around you come in to heal the wounds you feel. Also, you can sing Hu, as mentioned in the relaxation technique.

Now see if you still feel like eating something. Surprise! Unless you are truly hungry, after doing this sort of exercise, you probably won't have a desperate need to stuff something in your mouth.

External Authorities Begin to Take a Back Seat To Your Own Internal Authority

Some people let diets, weight-control centers, or nutritionists make all their decisions for them when they want to lose weight. Once you begin to take charge of your life through your creative imagination, you find that you are your own best authority when it comes to choosing the means and methods that are right for you. Of course there are well-educated and experienced experts to assist us in any field. You will know who to go to and what to do by following your own "internal authority".

Intuition is becoming more and more respected as a means to make decisions— when you combine it with good old-fashioned common sense. The two can be married to create a wonderful sense of self-reliance. With all the knowledge we have today about food, metabolism, exercise and psychology, we can conquer almost any weight-control problem by adding intuition, thinking thin, and a positive attitude. If just one important ingredient is missing, it may hold us back.

The way to be assured that we are doing everything we can is to continue to trust the inner authority, that higher self which is the true "image of God" we were made in. It will continue to guide us to what is best, regardless of what the "external authorities" may say. Remember to listen to it as you use your common sense.

Something You Can Do:

Take a moment now to write here or in your journal how you feel better about yourself and your own inner authority after thinking thin.

Thinking Thin Works As Long As you Choose to Use It

Danielle was aware of making healthier choices. She lost five pounds after her first week of thinking thin. She was listened to her inner authority and focused on her key image every morning and at night. When she awoke, she was aware of loving herself and seeing herself the way she used to be— lighter and happier. She kept the exercises near her bed and read a little bit of this book every day. Just doing these few simple things make her successful.

Linda took some time every morning to imagine her ideal image. She gets slimmer by the day, and her husband is handing out compliments she's never heard before!

Joannie used a key image and simply focused on it once a day in her meditation. She lost twenty pounds and two dress sizes.

The stories go on and on, but you can make your own. If you continue to think thin on a regular daily basis, you will prove to yourself, the most important person of all, that you do have the power to control your own life and your own body through focused imagination. In fact, you already do so.

Chapter 7

How to Spot Self-Sabotage

"The harder you fall, the higher you bounce."
— American Proverb

Whenever I really want something but can't seem to attain it, I know I am unconsciously holding myself back through my attitudes or old beliefs. Over and over again I have seen the impossible become possible, so why do I get in my own way?

The reasons often lie below the conscious level. How can we become aware of them and let them go? This chapter will help you remove any blocks you may run into while creating your new image. Through experience with many people, I have learned to spot certain signs that tell us when we're getting off track. Here are some of the most common ones, with some ideas to help you get back to thinking thin. Be creative in making up your own techniques, as well. Once you spot the cause of a problem, you're over halfway there to solving it. And as you know, whatever you believe will work certainly will!

Sign #1— You Hear Yourself Say, "This Isn't Working"

You may say to yourself, *"I'm gaining more weight."* I have done the same thing, so I know how easy it is to slip into old patterns of imagination. By now you're aware that worry and its companion images counteract the key image you are focusing on. It's a tired old record that plays over and over, even when you haven't gained weight at all.

No matter how much it seems that you are gaining weight (even if you *are*), the only thing that will ever *stop* that process and keep it from happening again is your commitment to thinking thin. In other words, you may feel you have lost the battle, but you *will win* the war by acting as if success is yours.

The influence of the subconscious on health is being expounded by medical experts everywhere. Some refer to neuro-peptides (protein-like brain molecules) in every cell of our body which are capable of changing themselves. That means every single cell in our bodies can "think". We are constantly renewing our own atom structure. (98% of your body was *not there* a year ago!) Consider how this ability of your body to respond to your thoughts can influence your body weight and health.

Since your body is actually a field of intelligence, doesn't it make sense that it will respond to your every thought and feeling? So how do you keep from worrying and bringing up old thought patterns? It is not always easy to do, but having a few simple "counter-attack" techniques helps.

Something You Can Do Now:

Identify any unwanted thought, action, or feeling. Imagine yourself mentally erasing it from the blackboard of your mind. Now replace it with a more desirable thought and feeling. Repeat the new, positive thought several times until you feel it inside.

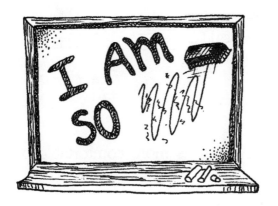

This exercise works because the mind is like a child. The old thought patterns are like familiar toys. The only way it will let go of the old thoughts (old toys) is by replacing them with new thoughts (new toys). That is exactly what you are doing with this exercise. It may need to be repeated often until the mind is able to let go of the old

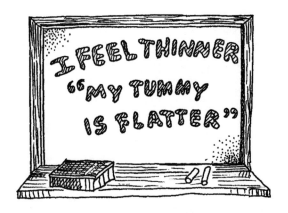

thoughts as it becomes more comfortable playing with new thoughts.

Sign # 2— You Feel Compelled To Weigh Yourself Often

We all fluctuate in weight by several pounds. You can weigh up to three or four pounds more at the end of the day than at the beginning. Weighing yourself may be your demise. It depressed me for weeks until I threw out my bathroom scales. Here is a simple exercise you can do to keep from weighing yourself and letting the scales influence your thoughts— instead of making new thoughts to influence the scales.

Something You Can Do Now:

Throw out your scales! (Unless you are under strict doctor's orders to weigh yourself).

It can't get simpler than that— and there is really no other answer. (If you wish, you can give them to a friend to keep for awhile, but *do not have them anywhere within your access.*) If your roommate or someone else in your family wants to use them, I would ask that they be hidden from you, at least for now. If you are concerned that you won't know if you are seriously gaining weight, don't worry, your clothes will tell you. Now erase that thought!

Sign #3— You Are Beating Yourself Over the Head For Thinking Negatively

Take heart! Guilt seems to be an integral part of most cultures, but is not necessary for our purposes. Not only is guilt unnecessary, it is very detrimental to your self-image. You may want to contemplate the positive effects of loving yourself thin.

Something You Can Do Now:

If you hear yourself saying things like, *"I shouldn't be thinking negatively"* or *"Thinking fat will not solve my problems, I am so dumb!"* Just say to yourself, *"stop!"*

Now replace the feelings of guilt with a feeling of love for yourself because you *are* taking steps to make your life better. You are doing the very best you can and every "thin" thought you have about the new you is another step in the right direction.

Sign #4— You Are Feeling Guilty for Eating Something You Think You Shouldn't Have Eaten

Do you think thin people feel guilty for eating certain foods? Not likely, unless they are going against a doctor's orders. No, thin people blithely eat whatever they feel like. Guess what? That's part of thinking thin!

I understand the feeling of eating something you wish you hadn't and then feeling guilty for it. I have had those feelings most of my life. I overcame them by telling myself that as long as I was going to go ahead and eat something sinful I would enjoy it totally. After I started thinking thin, I knew guilt would only hold me back by making me think there were things I "shouldn't eat."

Thinking thin means thinking that you *are* thin already. You are a slim person who can eat whatever she or he wants. You love and trust yourself totally, and can depend on your instinct to tell you what you need. You eat only until you are full and no more, even when there is a huge buffet in front of you, or a big holiday dinner. You may even leave food on your plate if you are too full to finish it! It is simply your way of life to regard food as nourishment and nothing more, unless you have some special interest in cooking.

If you do happen to eat too much, or regret a rich meal, you simply say to yourself, *"I do this so rarely. I really enjoyed it too."* Then go on about your life.

Making a big deal out of eating only makes it a more of a big deal to your subconscious, which makes your body respond by gaining weight. Here's a way to counteract that.

Something You Can Do Now:

When you feel like you are being hard on yourself about what you are eating, tell the "guilt manager" to lay off. In fact, fire her!   Now enjoy the next meal you eat, and say to yourself, *"everything I eat turns to energy!"* Tell yourself that even if you eat a lot, your body probably has to burn more calories than you ate to digest all that food! Go for a walk if possible, and breathe the fresh air. It will alleviate that "full" feeling, which may have contributed to feeling heavier as well as guilty.

Sign #5— You Find Yourself Listening to What Other People or the Media Say

It has really thrown me off at times to hear commercials that gave me the feeling I needed to change my body in order to change my image. In reality, it's the other way around. The image will never permanently change simply by changing the body. Especially when you're using a diet program or other outside stimulus as a crutch. The self-image has to improve at some point, so you can make a change in you body that will last a lifetime.

When other people talk about dieting, it is tempting to fall back into the pattern of thinking that food is the sole determiner of your weight. Of course it does have an impact, but why do people keep talking about dieting? Because for those who rely on it, a diet is a never-ending necessity to keep their weight down. Stay clear of those conversations whenever possible, for a clear head and the best results.

Also, others may view the quest for thinness as though it were the holy grail. Or they project this thought form on you. Your view of being healthy may be quite different from the average Jane's. You may feel that your body is most comfortable and attractive at a size 12 than a stick-figure 6 or 8. Why not have the kind of body you have decided you want, not what someone else thinks you should have?

The whole key to maintaining your own way of thinking while thinking thin is to become *your own authority.* You can decide exactly how you want to look— and then hold the image!

Something You Can Do Now:

Write here or in your journal what your ideal "look" is.

_____

Now decide that you have every right to look that way, no matter what other people or the media say is "correct". You are your own authority and you may just be the trend-setter for the next generation! Consider how vital a role that may be. Someone has to begin to break the pattern of conforming to unhealthy or unrealistic images. Why not you?

Sign #6— You Become Discouraged Due to Regaining Weight or Becoming Impatient

In some cases, including mine, you might actually gain weight after starting to think thin. There are very sound reasons for this. Sometimes you have to gain a little muscle in order to burn more calories. Muscle weighs more than fat! Or you may have to go up a little to balance your system before it starts to drop impurities and fat.

On the other hand, old thoughts and images may be making a last stand. This is good, because if forces them to surface so you can clean them out with new thoughts and images. Patience and persistence worked for me— and it can work for you too. We have been so inundated with the "instant results" promised in every department of life we may forget that high quality, lasting results depend upon generous amounts of love, energy, and time.

How many years have you been programmed to be overweight? If you think about how many hefty thoughts have gone into your subconscious over the years, you may get a *fraction* of an idea of what it may take to undo all that damage to your self image. You have the rest of your life to consciously think thin, so start now, before more unconsciously negative thought patterns creep in. You can overcome them with some time and love. After awhile, thinking thin becomes such a natural way of life you won't even have to try anymore. It will seem odd to think any other way. After twelve years of thinking thin, I've enjoyed ten of those *being* thin. How's that for results?

Something You Can Do:

If you find yourself gaining weight back, or becoming impatient about your progress, think of the following stories.

Arie Luyendyk thought of himself as a race car driver for *ten years*. He had a singular image of himself as a winner, even though he had never won a race. When other race car drivers traveled, drank, and vacationed after races, Arie went straight home to his strict schedule of health club workouts and gourmet cuisine. This was part of his discipline of thinking of himself as a winner. He focused on his ideal image and never gave up. Luyendyk finally fulfilled his image in a very big way. He won the 1990 Indianapolis 500 in the last few laps! All because he refused to give up. He was a winner inside, but it took a tremendous amount of patience— along with a very firm focus of attention— to manifest the outside reality.

If you are feeling discouraged, read stories of people who have had to overcome great odds to attain their goals. It won't be hard to find those kinds of stories because anyone who has become a success had done so at some cost.

I don't know many people who have walked into success through an open gate. The way is strewn with roadblocks for most, so be patient with yourself and the process if you really want success. It also helps to know that those roadblocks are easily surmountable with the tools given in this book.

There May Be Subconscious Reasons For Retaining Extra Weight

As I began to "think myself thin," I was receptive to the suggestions from my subconscious that would help me take the weight off. I looked for the inner reasons I had retained the weight. I embarked on a psychological safari through my own inner being, to discover why I had chosen to be so heavy. From my explorations and those of many others, I have discovered some common reasons for carrying extra weight.

As you begin the imaginative process of seeing yourself thin, refer back to this chapter from time to time to see if one or more of these reasons may apply to your particular situation.

Reason #1— Self-Protection

Extra weight can act as a protective barrier to shield the individual from someone or something. This is distrust of one's own inner strength. People have often told me that they felt like victims, or felt insecure and unsure of having enough love in their life. This was sometimes reflected back to them by others in the form of criticism, rejection, or mistreatment of some kind.

These feelings are sometimes caused by low self-esteem, common to many of us. Feeling inadequate or weak can be overcome with some effort by loving yourself more. If you could see the spiritual being that you are, you'd know that there is no need to protect yourself from life, your own choices, or others' disapproval. You are connected to all things and all life.

Something You Can Do Now:

Find a comfortable spot to sit quietly for a few minutes with pen and paper. Relax with a few deep breaths and think about the situations that may make you feel protective of your feelings. Write down the first one that comes to mind.

Ask yourself why you feel the way you do and how you might change those feelings. It may be talking with the people involved, trusting yourself more, loving yourself more, or simply taking charge of your life.

Write a note to yourself under the place where you wrote the situation. Tell yourself you will take care of this situation and describe how and when you will do so. Then sign and date it, just as if you were making a contract with yourself. Now the means to resolve it can become clear to you through your subconscious.

Feelings of self-protection may also come from a real need to leave a situation or change it. Good psychological counseling can be helpful in resolving weight problems associated with these issues, particularly if you are having difficulty resolving them on your own.

Reason #2— Carrying a Burden

Some people "carry the weight" of their problems or the burdens of others. Those who tend to be "worriers" or feel responsible for everyone else may try to help by "carrying the load."

Sandy realized that the more successful her business became, the more weight she gained! She needed to delegate to other people as more work came in. As soon as she recognized this cause for her weight and started trusting her coworkers more, she improved her self-image and she dropped the pounds.

Something You Can Do Now:

Sit in a comfortable chair with pen and paper handy. Close your eyes and breathe deeply for a few moments, relaxing every part of your body.

Now look within yourself and ask your higher self or God to show you what kind of burden you may be carrying. Write it down. Take a look at the burden and ask yourself how you can "redistribute the weight" of this responsibility back to the individual or universe. Let God take care of it!

Last, let go of all responsibility that is not yours by imagining it as an extra amount of water in your body that simply flows out like a waterfall from you.

This may require professional counseling. It is an individual choice. You will know if and when it is necessary for you simply by keeping your attention riveted to your ideal image.

Reason #3— Filling an Unfilled Need

The old "fix it with an ice cream cone" syndrome is common to many of us. Many people have been raised on the idea that sweets or rich food would take care of everything from a tummy ache to a heart ache. It's the old food-equals-love syndrome. If we don't feel we are getting enough love, we often try to replace the emptiness inside with food.

Something You Can Do:

As before, find a quiet place to rest for a moment and relax your entire body. Imagine a golden fountain pouring forth the most delectable water in the universe. It is so satisfying that no earthly water can touch it. It is really God's love for you, and you can fill yourself with as much as you want! Now you are so full with this love that you have lots to give out to others. Find something you can do to help someone else today. Visit a friend who is lonely, smile at the people at the supermarket, or get started on that volunteer work you have been meaning to do. Place your attention outside yourself.

Again, if the situation seems to be out of hand, look within yourself and see if you may feel guided to receive professional help. There may be a support group that can help you. Check the phone book and newspapers to see if something nudges you in the right direction.

Just keep seeing yourself the way you wish to be, no matter what you are eating, and either you will become a more balanced eater, or you will find help in replacing love for food.

Reason #4— You Have Difficulty Saying No

Some experts say that people who are overweight have difficulty saying "no," and that when they learn to express how they feel and act on it, they lose weight. Julie had trouble saying "no" to her adult children. They each had families of their own, but were relying on her a little more than they should. When her son's family moved in with her, she had trouble losing the weight she was carrying for them.

Are you always helping others without taking time for yourself? Are you surrounded by people who need things from you? Then you may be someone who needs to learn to say "no". I had this problem. I still watch myself to make sure I don't take on projects or responsibilities, no matter how small, if they don't feel right.

Something You Can Do Now:

Next time someone asks you to do something, try saying, "Let me think about it." Then give yourself the respect you would give anyone else! Take time to decide if it really is something you want to do. You might see if there are classes or workshops on assertiveness training that may help support your efforts to love yourself enough to take care of yourself.

Reason #5— Avoiding Facing Fears or Other Blocks to Success

A mythical woman we'll call Sally had been hurt so much that she unconsciously decided to guard herself against further hurt. She did this by becoming so unattractive it seemed to her no one could love her.

It started with weight gain, the quickest way for the subconscious to respond to her unconscious desire to be ugly. Then she wondered if it was worth it to even attempt to look pretty. She let herself go. Over time, her self-image took a real beating.

This downward spiral can trap anyone who has given up hope. If you find yourself wanting love, but not wanting to risk the pain, you *can* do something about it.

Something You Can Do

Loving yourself as much as possible is the key to becoming free. You will no longer depend on someone else to love you or be devastated if they don't. You can become self-contained. This subject is covered in many good books, and can be helped by a good counselor.

Also, you can read my booklet, *How to Love Yourself, So Others Can Love You More* (available through any bookstore).

For now, here is an exercise you can do daily to fill yourself with love.

Simply hug yourself and tell yourself that you love you and will take care of you for your entire life, in the best way possible. Promise to treat yourself like a precious jewel. This is almost like a wedding ceremony, because it is a commitment to yourself. It is very real and it feels very good!

One woman who does this every day found her clothes getting bigger and bigger and her skin feeling like silk!

Reason #6— Someone Else Wants You to Lose Weight

Is it truly you, the *real you*, that wants to lose weight, or someone *else* who holds a thinner image of you? A loved one may feel you should have a different size or shape. *Maybe you really feel fine just the way you are!* If you accept someone else's image, you are allowing them to control you. This is giving away your personal power to be an individual, free expression of life.

Something You Can Do Now:

See the self-image exercise at the end of Chapter 1, on creating your own ideal self image. Do this exercise now using the feelings *you* have about how you would like to look and feel. Watch to see if your descriptions are your own or something you have heard someone else say.

"Being yourself" sounds simple, but it is really a continual learning and unfolding process that takes a lifetime. Being patient with yourself will help to keep you on track.

There Are Many Ways to Resolve Problems, Deadlocks, and Resistance as There Are Other People:

The Easiest, Simplest Thing You Can Do to Remove Blocks to Success is to Simply Maintain Your Focus on the Key Image You Have Created.

This brief list of difficulties is by no means a complete. Whatever your reasons for retaining weight, you will discover your own ways to resolve them if you practice the exercises in this book faithfully. The subconscious works like a heat-seeking missile. It will draw to you the desired result by *whatever means it takes, as long as you continue to give it commands* in the form of images.

Be confident that you will attract whatever tools, help, or solutions needed to resolve your own special, unique and individual health issue. You can speed up this process by listening very carefully to your body's true wants and needs (unless of course you are already on a special diet under medical supervision). Listen to your "inner self" as it directs your actions, lights up someone's words regarding a particular nutritionist, allergist, exercise plan, or meditation program. There are almost as many reasons for retaining weight as there are people, so you will need to be receptive to your own inner direction.

Dreams Can Be Wonderful Tools for Removing Stumbling Blocks

If you are not sure you even have a subconscious reason for retaining weight, you can use this method:

Just before going to sleep, write a note to your higher self, or to God. Ask for a dream that will show you *clearly* what your block may be to success in staying slim. In the morning, pick up the pen or pencil by your bedside and begin to write underneath the note written to God, "I remember dreaming about..." and write down *whatever* word or words come to mind, *even if they seem to have no meaning*. It is like a string of pearls. The first word (pearl) will pull out all the rest! Do this over and over again until you get some results.

Next, write under the dream words, "I know the meaning of this dream. It is... " Then write *whatever* comes to mind, no matter how silly it may seem.

One time I dreamed I could not get home because all the roads were blocked off. They were all under construction. Then one of the workers told me I could go a different way. The way he showed me was normally blocked, but was now open. I had to be flexible and look for other avenues, perhaps even pathways that did not work before, but could work for me now. I explored some new ideas for eating and exercise that came my way that week, and they worked wonders!

Do you believe in guardian angels? If you do, why not ask your guardian angel for help as you do these dream exercises? Some people report fantastic dreams or insights just by asking for help!

An Ounce of Prevention is Worth a Pound of Cure

If you want to prevent self-sabotage, try one or more of the following methods to keep yourself on track during the sensitive first few days, weeks, or months of thinking thin.

Method #1— Turn Your Attention Outward With Service

Most people find when they are very busy with activities they feel good about, they don't think about themselves as much. They think more about the project they are working on instead of their own problems. If you've ever volunteered at a hospice or hot line, you might actually become grateful for your own good fortune simply to be alive.

Try getting busy with service to your family, the handicapped, elderly folks, your church or religious organization, or an environmental group. It can be anything you love— that does not involve food or dieting!

Method #2— Watch Less Television

Television often brings weight increase through negative conditioning. It makes people focus on negative images or feel that they will never be good enough just as they are. TV makes it seem like we all need to smell, feel, and look better. At the same time, we are bombarded with commercials that tempt us to eat more and more unhealthy foods. Studies show teens who watch a lot of TV weigh more. They are less active and more likely to overindulge. The same can be said of adults.

Method #3— Being Creative is Thin Fun

Being artistic or creative in some way will also give the mind something to do besides criticize you for how you look. You will be focusing attention on creating beauty outside of yourself, which cannot help but make you feel more beautiful inside .

If you do not already have a hobby, check with your local community college. There are always courses on things like pottery, drawing, photography, folk dancing (great fun and great exercise), music, or art appreciation. Think of something you have always wanted to try, and prove to yourself how enjoyable it really is! Almost any skill or appreciation is simple to learn with patience and practice. These can be applied to thinking thin as well. Anything worthwhile and lasting takes time and (fun) effort.

Method #4— Dress To Feel Thin

Wear clothing that is not tight, but loose fitting and comfortable. Dress so that *you* feel attractive and *smaller* than your clothes.

Whenever you feel lost or confused, unsure of yourself and your ability to make this process work, look to whatever spiritual guidance you believe in and ask for help. Know that it will come. There are a million and one ways to resolve these issues and to lose weight, but it is up to you to find what works best for you. The means will present themselves as you maintain your vision and feeling of the goal accomplished. Relax and enjoy the process, as if you are playing a game. Sit back and watch the show and you will be amazed at the shape of things to come!

Chapter 8

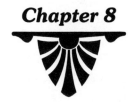

How to Form a Thinking Thin Support Group

"Be curious always, for knowledge will not acquire you, you must acquire it."
— Sadie Buck

Diet Programs Which Involve Support Are More Successful

Groups like Weight Watchers_ have many members because they provide a strong support system that dieting alone does not afford. Thinking Thin support groups have elicited comments like, "It helped keep my mind and attention on the focus," and "We talked about issues related to weight. It helped a lot!"

This chapter will show you when and how to form a support group of people who feel the same way you do and who can help you reach your goals.

Many women don't feel confident that they can reduce their weight unaided or alone. It doesn't surprise me that by now people feel they need more help, since every diet seems to end in more weight regained.

The most successful diet programs today are ones where people receive emotional as well as dietary support. The role of self-image in weight management is becoming more widely recognized in the 1990's. I believe the greatest success will come when people learn how to change their self-image first. That's what a thinking thin support group is all about.

I once knew a woman who had cancer and joined a support group. She had lost hope, even though her husband tried to encourage her and give her strength. The group gave her the insight, through others' successes, to see how she could reach a new rung on the ladder of health. They shared key attitudes and thoughts that had helped them overcome cancer. The woman began to visualize her own recovery as she met others who had beat their own illness. She made it through and later even had a child, which she had been told was impossible. Support groups can provide powerful medicine for body, mind, and soul!

There Are Ways To Tell If the "Buddy System" Is For You Now

The following signals may tell you that a support group can be of some benefit to you now:

Signal #1— You Are Feeling Alone in This New Way of Thinking

Perhaps there is no one in your immediate circle of friends or family to support or believe in you and your thinking thin process. It may be that you feel more comfortable keeping it quiet right now among your family and friends. You believe in thinking thin, but you are not sure anyone else in your family will support it just yet.

Signal #2— You Don't Quite Believe This Can Work For You

You want to believe thinking thin will work and you want to make it work, but you are not quite convinced. You want to see it work for other people first. Perhaps you just want to hear other people say *they* believe thinking thin is a very real solution.

Signal #3— You Want to Speed Up the Process

You are aware there is strength in numbers. You know that the process will go faster with a group meeting weekly which will keep your attention riveted to your goal.

Signal #4— You Want the Support of Others Who Are In the Same Boat

This is a simple case of human nature. We all feel better when we know someone else has the same problem. From there, we can help each other reach the best solutions with compassion and understanding.

Signal #5— You Want to Be Reinforced By Others' Success

When you see this process working for other people, it may reinforce and strengthen your own resolve. You will feel motivated to become just as successful.

Signal #6— You Want to Be of Service By Helping Others Be Successful

This last signal indicates that you are well on your way to success yourself, because you are completing the circle by being of service to others. It is a universal principle that whatever you do comes back to you. Therefore, the service you give others in becoming more of what they want to be will allow you to become more of what you want to be.

Building Your Own Private Support Group is Easy and Simple

I would like to make it as easy as possible for you to begin your own support group. Here are a few simple clues I can give you to begin, and then you can be as creative as you like on your own.

Attitude is the Most Important Key to Beginning Any Endeavor

As in signal #7, wanting to be of service to others as well as yourself is the greatest attitude to begin with. It speaks of love for yourself and your fellow human beings in their attempts to reach greater heights.

I know the more I give to this project, helping people see their own inherent ability to control their lives, the more control I have over my own life, health and well-being. My attitude must be one of service with love, or I simply don't get the results I would like in my own life!

Set Your Goals For the Group You Want

Remember how we talked about writing down goals in the beginning of the book? It works well to help bring about the desired result. Think now about what kind of group you would like to have. What would be an ideal number of people? Where would you like to meet? What day and time would you like to meet? What kind of atmosphere would you like to create (welcoming, warm, educational)? Write your answers here:

Number of people _____

When _____

Where _____

Atmosphere _____

Find Your Meeting Place First

Using the thinking thin principles of focused imagination, find your meeting place by first imagining what kind of setting you would like to meet in. It could be someone's home, a bank meeting room, or church where you can make a small donation for the use of the room.

Make some phone calls to find out what is available. If you want to meet in someone's home, you may find a volunteer among those in your support group. Or you may choose to alternate homes for your meetings. Some groups who work together meet after hours at a restaurant to talk about thinking thin, and enjoy eating guilt-free!

Talk to Friends Who You Feel Would Be Receptive to the Idea

Once you have an idea of where and when you want to meet, you will sound much more organized and serious when talking with friends about establishing a support group.

You probably know which friends or associates would be receptive to the ideas found in thinking thin. Ask them to read the book *How to Think Yourself Thin* and tell you what they think. They can order this through any bookstore or through the 1-800 line listed in the back of this book. (Don't loan out your copy of this book— it's your only support right now. Hang on to it.)

Have an Initial Meeting to Discuss and Agree Upon Details

Meet at least once with your core group of friends, associates, and acquaintances who are interested in a thinking thin support group. Ask them:

1. If the time and place you have chosen are agreeable, and how often you would like to meet. I would suggest once a week minimum, for best results. Set up a certain number of weeks (eight is a good number), and ask people to commit to coming for eight weeks to test it.

2. Who would like to lead the first session (unless you choose to lead it yourself). You may appoint a group leader or share the leadership by alternating leaders for each meeting. Please note the suggested sample outlines for support group meetings at the end of this chapter. Anyone can follow the simple plan.

3. How long your meetings should last (put a limit on them, or they can go on forever!) I would suggest one hour; don't let it run more than one and one half hours.

4. How much they would like to donate for the service they are receiving. The amount isn't important but the principle is, as people will always get more out of service if they have paid something for it. They will also value it more highly.

I would suggest $2.00 to $5.00 per person per class. The money can go to renting a meeting room, copying extra materials, buying or renting inspirational materials such as video tapes, audio tapes, or books on positive thinking and visualization. I suggest appointing a treasurer or bookkeeper for the group. Involve as many people who want to be of service in some aspect of the group, for a firmer base of support.

5. What are the goals of the group? They can be to support the members in thinking thin, learn how to love oneself more, become healthier, develop inner strength, gain a greater self-image, help others feel good about themselves, improve the member's overall quality of life, or any goals you set as a group.

Even If You Only Know One Other Person Who Wants to Meet, It Is Enough

It's perfectly O.K. and beneficial for just two people to meet and support each other in the thinking thin process. Two people together are much stronger than two people alone. A team of two horses can pull a much heavier load, so team up and get rid of that load!

If you are too busy, immobile, or unable for any reason to physically meet with others, try a telephone-buddy system. Arrange to call someone once a week or more to stay in touch with each other's progress. You can still use the outline at the end of this chapter to structure the phone calls. Encourage a friend to increase their understanding of life with you and you will find yours expanding even more quickly.

You May Feel a Support Group is Not For You

I did this process all by myself, because no one had ever heard of thinking thin years ago! I was afraid my friends would think I had gone completely nuts if I even mentioned it. Now, of course, people are much more open to the idea of a mind-body connection.

Nonetheless, I was successful completely on my own, with large doses of patience, persistence, and self-discipline. I had to be my own best friend through all that time and I am now more confident in my own ability to create my own world because of it.

I do think I may have moved more quickly into the new me if I had been able to find the support of others. But if outer groups are not for you, don't hesitate to go it alone. Or you might try imagining an inner group of supportive friends, favorite heroes, and relatives who cheer on your efforts. Make it fun!

Support Groups Help Because They Keep Your Attention Focused

Doris loaned her copy of *How to Think Yourself Thin* to a friend for a few weeks, and found her success diminishing, because she had lost her link to the ideas. Joanne went on vacation and lost her focus, finding herself backsliding into old patterns. When they joined support groups, they both exclaimed how wonderful it was to have help thinking thin. Thoughts are powerful, but sometimes ephemeral. They can come and go quickly, leaving us in old ruts of self-images and habits.

Many people have written to say that support groups keep the minds and attention focused on thinking thin, because they are either reflecting on the meeting of just a day or two ago or looking forward to the meeting coming up. When you know the group is going to meet every week, you keep your key image in your conscious mind more often.

Doris found the exchange of examples on how the subconscious was helping her friends lose weight very inspirational. Joanne found the group made her feel good about herself. Everyone in the group agreed to think of each other in a positive, slim light.

Cindy felt the main benefit of her thinking thin group was the exploration of issues relating to weight. The group touched on many different physical, emotional, mental, and social reasons for retaining extra pounds. She found her own reason for being heavy in these discussions, and was able to consciously let it go.

Leading a Support Group Is Easy With the Proper Tools

Use the class outlines below to begin a support group. Later, the formats can be adapted to your particular group's needs and interests. But for the first month, stick with the topics given here, to keep the dynamics of thinking thin flowing. You may already have experience in leading support groups, and your ideas will flourish as you integrate the key ideas into new group activities and discussions.

Practice one of the exercises in this book at each weekly meeting until you run out, then start all over again. Repetition is a vital part of learning, so feel at ease using the same exercises again after a month or two. You may also ask the group each week what creative exercises and techniques for the subconscious that they have come up with. Everyone can contribute to the group. In fact, that is what makes support meetings such exciting opportunities for growth!

Tools For Leading a Dynamic Support Group

Tool #1— Always Start Out on a Positive, Happy Note

Laying a foundation of trust is vital for nurturing an open group discussion. That trust is created when people feel good, when their hearts are open. Start by having the group share how successful they have been already. Then they won't feel so bad talking about things that may not have gone so well.

Make sure the group knows the format of beginning on a positive note and why. Trust that the people in your group are there because they are intelligent, open-minded beings or they would not even be interested!

The best way to start on a happy note is to ask each person to share a success in the past week. It certainly does not have to be about weight management or food! It might be a new assignment at work, a vacation, or an insight from a child. Food topics, in fact, should be avoided completely. Everyone will have strong and different approaches to eating, and there is no need for comparison among the group. Thinking thin is about attitudes and images, not specific actions, and *definitely* not about food!

So start by asking, "What happened this week that made you feel successful, even just a little? Was it at work, at home, in thinking thin, or during your free time? What made the success happen?"

After each individual shares her success, the group can take a moment to reflect on the principles of how and why successes happen. They might ask the group member how she thought before and after the success. How did he or she feel? Explore the ingredients to feeling good about oneself.

Tool #2— Expressing Fears and Concerns is Also Essential

Allowing people to express their innermost thoughts and feelings about their weight, eating habits, and how they think people view them is vital to healing old, painful images. When a supportive, loving environment is provided, the best healer is to simply listen to each other.

Listening allows the individual to discover her own answers. This is how we all learn the most lasting lessons, of course. If one of the members is stuck on a problem, encourage the group to listen and express how they might handle the same obstacle.

One of the "ground rules" for your meeting is that anyone can ask for help and advice, or simply supportive listening. Not everyone will want help; some people will just want to share their struggles without comment. Encourage members to articulate what they need from the group at the moment to promote the greatest learning and the quickest results.

Tool #3— Ask How They Overcame Limiting Thoughts and Images

Be sure to find out how sad experiences were resolved, or negative thoughts were overcome. This brings you back around to the positive again, so everyone feels good and knows there is always a way out. Ask people with unresolved problems, "How would you handle this situation in some other area of your life? If you were at work, what would you do?" If they are at a loss, ask, "Would you mind letting someone else make suggestions?" Then ask the group if anyone has an idea to resolve the issue.

Tool #4— Bring Out a Principle of Success in Thinking Thin

Choose one specific principle or chapter to discuss each time you meet. Explore together how you have each already been successful with that specific principle in other areas of life.

For example: Relaxation is an important principle to use before trying to use the imagination.

Ask the group, "How has relaxation helped you in accomplishing goals in your life? What role does it play in getting things done?"

Next, create an exercise for homework involving that principle. It can be the one in Chapter 5, or one you or other class members make up. Challenge the class to do the exercise once a day for the next week.

Tool #5— Writing Can Be Healing and Insightful

Ask each member of the group to bring their copy of *How to Think Yourself Thin* and their thinking thin journal to each meeting. If you like, you can buy special class journals from the funds received for the sessions.

As the group members talks, give people a chance to write down answers and insights in their books or journals. Some people will be hesitant to talk out loud, so writing in their journal gives them a chance to express themselves without talking. The more the class members write, the greater their understanding will become.

The journal will provide a vehicle for people to chart their own progress and realizations throughout the time they are struggling to escape the cocoon of old thought patterns. Ask them to review it daily for inspiration and support.

Tool #6— Ask Everyone Who Joins the Group to Re-read This Chapter Before They Attend

If you all read this chapter, you'll meet on common ground and be able to pool your best ideas for a dynamic, uplifting group.

Tool #7— You Can Use the Following Outline to Lead a Successful Support Group

Outline For Thinking Thin Support Groups

1. Ask each person to *share the positive experiences* they had during the week (or since you last met). Ask them to record their experience in their journals now.

Ask the individual members to explore the times they had success with changing their thoughts and images. It could have been an experience that left them feeling good about themselves, or a time when a dream came true.   Emphasize thoughts and images or success in all areas not necessarily relating to food and weight. Eating healthy and being the shape you want to be are a natural result of how you think about yourself. Food talk, i.e., what they ate or did not eat this week, should be ruled out unless it relates to how new thoughts and images created new desires and habits.

2. Ask everyone to *write down their present fears, concerns, or setbacks* in thinking about or imagining a new figure.

Ask for ideas on how they can resolve these issues and overcome the limiting thoughts. If a group member is stuck, ask if she would like the group to brainstorm new approaches to the problem. Or ask her to explore how she would tackle the same problem in another setting, i.e. at work, in her relationship, or at home.

3. Bring out one *new principle* from the weekly assigned chapter for everyone to discuss. Ask the group to write down how they have already been successful with this principle in some area of their lives.

Now ask them to discuss how they plan to apply it to thinking themselves thin.

4. Give a *creative exercise* using that same principle. Do the exercise together right now for practice. Ask if there are any questions and let the group answer.

5. Give *homework*. Assign the above exercise to the group to practice once a day. Ask them to jot down their results to share next week.

A thinking thin support group can be a very enjoyable learning experience. Many people form lasting friendships and find a new approach to all areas of their lives. I have seen group members release unwanted careers or abusive relationships, take control of their lives, and become svelte and confident as they practice the universal principles found in thinking thin. A support group can be a tremendous service to those who are ready to take a next step in life. Leading a thinking thin support group will boost your own efforts tenfold!

I welcome your comments, suggestions, or questions regarding support groups. Here's to your continued success!

Chapter 9

Maintaining the New You

"Measure wealth not by the things you have, but by the things you have for which you would not take money."

— Anonymous

Does a garden still need watering after the first harvest? Won't it continue to yield food all by itself? Of course not! A garden needs constant attention as long as you wish it to remain beautiful. Pulling weeds, trimming plants, adding fertilizer, and watering are all necessary to maintain the status quo of your beautiful self-image garden.

The constant upkeep of desirable thoughts and images is an on-going part of maintaining your new slim self. The best way to accomplish this is by making it a habit. Anything done for twenty-eight days becomes second nature. Why not discipline yourself to carefully watch your thoughts and images regarding your body for a month and see how much easier it is after that?

Everything in Life Goes Backward or Forward— Nothing is Static

There are only two directions to go with your physical, emotional, mental and spiritual health: backward or forward. There is no in-between ground! In order to continue forward, becoming more and more healthy and more of what you want, it is vital to keep practicing the art of thinking thin. I did the exercises at the same time each day, until they became such a part of me that I didn't even have to think about them.

Now I think like a thin person— because I am a thin person— because I think like a thin person! I am at the chicken-or-the-egg point where I don't know which comes first. I just keep living life with the assumption that I am a thin person who can eat whatever she wants for health whenever she wants, so I do! These days, I also try to make sure I eat enough because *I don't want to lose weight!* Does this sound like someone with forty extra pounds who dieted off and on for twelve years?

Gratitude is Key to Maintaining Your Weight and Shape

Is the glass half empty or half full? Do you feel grateful for your weight loss, or are you still comparing yourself to movie stars? Whenever I feel grateful for what I have, it seems to perpetuate and create more health and abundance. Being grateful for how you look and feel will improve your state of mind as well as your appearance.

A universal principle is at work whenever people count their blessings. Remember the principle of self-acceptance—that you have to feel fine about yourself before you can get slim? Over and over again, I have observed that people who relax and appreciate themselves as they are release weight easily. So perpetuate the process by remembering to be grateful for the new you!

If I catch myself thinking I am gaining weight, I immediately replace those thoughts with ones like *"I feel so thin!"* and *"I am so grateful for being where I am now, forty pounds lighter than I was twelve years ago!"*

Replace *"I still feel heavy"* with *"I'm so happy that I am slimmer!"*
Replace *"I'm still pear shaped"* with *"I'm thankful for feeling so much lighter!"*

Replace *"I wish I didn't have these saddlebags"* with *"Look how much progress I've made!"*

Something You Can Do Now:

Write down a limiting thought that you have been holding about yourself. Now replace it with one that is upbuilding and grateful.

Thoughts Affect Your Future

Even if you have already attained the new you, more thoughts about the old you will go into your seed pile and eventually sprout if they are not cut off at the root! No matter how wealthy, healthy or wise we are, imagination is the reigning force in our manifesting subconscious. Not one of us can escape its effects, not even a spiritual giant. So consciously choose the seeds you want to grow in your new garden.

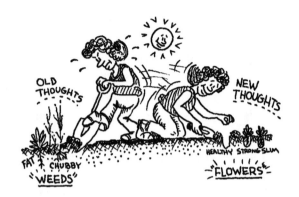

Release Fear, Worry, and Other Emotions Regarding Weight

Fear is a mighty motivator for the imagination. Have you every worried that something would happen— and then it did? I began gaining weight when I was young simply because I feared it. The only solution I have found is to replace the unconscious negative emotion with a positive one as soon as I am aware of it.

Avoid the *"What if I gain the weight back?"* syndrome by feeling grateful. Fear and thankfulness do not mix! Choose the feelings you want to hold about yourself.

Something You Can Do Now:

If you ever feel heavier, whether it is due to water weight, shrunken clothes or any other reason:

1. Tell yourself, "Oh that's just temporary, it will go away soon."

2. Wear loose clothing during low ebbs. This will help take your attention off your body.

3. Now get busy with something you enjoy doing. Help someone else, tackle a tough project, or start a new hobby— and keep thinking thin!

To Keep Moving Forward, Set New Goals Right Away

My sisters always said our family had "pot bellies" and that I simply had to hold my stomach in! Once I realized I could use my imagination to become thinner, I decided to try reshaping my body. It worked! I have accepted the fact that my body will never be perfect, for whose body ever is? But I have been able to effect some minor adjustments that make me feel more confident about my ability to be in control of my life. My tummy is much flatter now than it was before, because now I *know* I can change my life via my imagination.

As soon as you begin to see the results of your thinking thin efforts (don't wait until you are "there"), make new images that improve your shape, health, strength, and energy even more. What else would you like to change?

Something You Can Do Now:

1. Write here or in your journal one thing you are still complaining about in regard to your body shape or health habits:

_____

2. Look at what you wrote, and write here or in your journal what you would like instead:

_____

3. Make up a key image for it. (For example, my key image for a flat stomach was the new fit of my leotards and tights when I danced):

_____

4. Now make up a key phrase to go with your key image (for example, *"I have a nice, flat stomach"*).

_____

Every time you get down on yourself about the complaint in part one of this exercise, replace it with the key image in part three and the key phrase in part four.

Continuing To Improve Other Areas of Body Image Assumes You Have Reached Your Goal

By making new goals for yourself right now, just after you have begun to see some results from thinking thin, you are using a very powerful principle. It works just like climbing a ladder. How will you get up the ladder if you can't see the next rung? You are actually creating each rung as you go, so it's important to focus upward and set your next health goal now.

Setting up new images convinces the subconscious mind that you have indeed attained the desired results from your first goal. It's kind of a trick that you can play on yourself to ensure success. The mind loves to finish one cycle before it begins the next. And it loves to know what is coming down the road for it to work on. Setting new goals will help you complete the new cycle of your first goal in the most expedient manner— by assuming it is done.

Are You Accepting The New You?

How do you hold and carry yourself? Are you standing tall and proud or slouching like you are still trying to hide something about your appearance? Pamela hasn't reached her goal yet, but even so, she wears her blouses tucked in and stands up straight, proud and tall. She thinks and acts like a thin person and I never think of her as overweight. Pamela just exudes confidence in how she looks, because she imagines herself thin. *She is already focused on maintenance.*

Years ago I had people compliment me on my weight loss, or how thin I looked, when I did not have the confidence to know I looked good yet. Because I did not yet believe I was thin, it was more of a struggle to keep the weight off. I finally began to accept the compliments and see that I had indeed become thinner.

Changing the "Core Image" Will Change Your Life Forever

"I can eat whatever I want, whenever I want to." That's my battle cry and has been for years. I had granola last night at nine p.m. This morning I ate watermelon for breakfast. I eat what my body needs when it needs it. I am a thin person and that is how I will stay, no matter what I do! Of course, by thinking this way, I will do what is best for my body to maintain that healthy image.

Something You Can Do Now:

Imagine yourself right now eating whatever you want, whenever you want to, for the rest of your life.

1. Make up a key image here of yourself refusing your favorite desert simply because you can have it any time you want and you have had enough of it for now. For example, I no longer crave cheesecake, which I used to love, because I rarely desire rich foods anymore. However, when I want them, I eat them with relish.

Write here or in your journal what your new image is:

_____

2. Make up a key phrase that exemplifies your greatest desire in terms of being a thin person, whether it is eating whatever you want, wearing whatever you want, or doing a favorite sport or activity. Remember to phrase this in the positive. Instead of writing, *"I don't have to wear tent dresses anymore,"* write, *"I can wear form-fitting, flattering clothing."* Write your key phrase here:

_____

Stay in Touch With the Basic Principle of Imagination as Controller

Really, you are the controller of your images. The imagination is only a tool for you to use when you are aware of how it works.

Something You Can Do Now:

Reread this book with a highlighter or pencil. Mark the ideas and exercises you feel apply to you most. When you are feeling at a low point with regard to your self-image, re-read your highlights and your favorite exercises.

Try reading other inspiring books as well, in order to stay on track. See the suggested reading list for ideas, or ask your local librarian for inspiring grist for your image mill!

Chapter 10

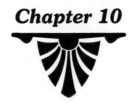

Beyond Thinking Thin

"When you aim for perfection, you discover it's a moving target."

— George Fisher

What happens after you become the size and shape you want? Now that you are free of the burden you have been carrying, you can shift your attention to something else. The mind is like a child who always needs to have something to do, because that is its nature. In order to keep it occupied with something other than old patterns, it is important to give it a new goal on which to focus.

As soon as I discovered just how powerful my imagination was in changing my body, I reached out to other areas of life that needed changing. Surprise! I discovered that I could think my stomach flatter, think my hips trimmer, and even think myself younger. As always, nothing is ever perfect, but the changes in my life have been most dramatic.

I am making tremendous progress in all areas of my life by investing in my imagination. I even took a course from a company called "Executive Futures" that showed me how to focus on success via the imagination and relaxing the nervous system daily. People who are successful in any endeavor in life are aware of the importance of imagination and use it for *everything*.

You may have heard of a book called *Pyschocybernetics* by Maxwell Malt. He describes many tests that prove the power of the imagination. One such group was practicing throwing darts. The control group practiced hitting the target every day. The test group only practiced in their minds, by visualizing hitting the target. Both groups did equally well. It is interesting to note, however, that those who practiced physically hitting the target in addition to visualization came out way ahead of either group!

Imagine Your Next Dream Now

While continuing to think about and imagine your new self-image, try a few small experiments in other areas of your life. These can be as simple as re-decorating a room or as challenging as redirecting your career or lifestyle. It doesn't matter how you start, as it will prove to you once more that you really are in charge of your life.

Jackie decided to apply the principles of thinking thin to creating a new relationship. Twice a day, she focused on the perfect relationship. She imagined specific values, activities, and ideals she and her partner would share. Using her imagination, she conjured up the kind of lifestyle they would enjoy and the good qualities her partner would have. They would give each other lots of space to grow. She wanted someone who cherished her as much as she cherished him and who had the strength to show her that love.

The most important aspect of her visualization, she told me, was to see it all as a game. The visualization was a game, and she imagined herself and her new partner playing a new game of life together. She kept it light and neutral, not desperate.

Jackie then opened her heart and told God she was ready for the right man in her life. Soon afterward, she told me that she already knew her future husband— he had just been revealed to her in a new light! Jackie and her new fianc_ had been the best of friends for a long time. She just had to open herself to something more in her own life. They have been happily married now for some time.

Something You Can Do Now:

Write down an area of your life you would like to improve. If you are not sure where to begin, look at the list I've supplied here and see if anything jumps out at you.

Relationships
Finance
Health
Career
Family
Children
Friendships
Spirituality
Education
Hobbies
Creativity
Home/House
Vacations
Time Management

After choosing an area to work on, write here or in your journal what your ideal would be for that area of your life. Make it as detailed as possible.

Now create a key image for your dream. An example would be if you want a new home, see yourself unlocking the front door to your new house with a sigh of contentment. Walk in and see it decorated just the way you like. Remember to use all the senses possible: smell, sounds, taste, touch, emotion, and thoughts. Describe your key image for your chosen area of change here:

Create a key phrase for your new dream. Think of a short sentence to describe what you want as if you already have it. For example, *"I have a gorgeous new house and I am so grateful for it!"* Remember to use only positive words. Leave out all the no's, don'ts, or won'ts. Write your key phrase here:

As in thinking thin, it is vital to focus daily on your most desired goals. Choose a time you can focus on this particular goal, key image and key phrase. If you can do it twice a day, so much the better. Be sure to relax using the methods in Chapter 5 before you focus, or just take a few deep breaths, releasing any stress before you work with your key image and phrase. It is best to choose a quiet time in the morning upon awakening or in the evening before going to sleep where you can spend a few minutes focusing on several goals you may have. If that is impossible, try making a deal with yourself to do this every time you brush your teeth, make your bed, or shower, and you will definitely reap the rewards.

If Others Can Do It, You Can Do It Too!

I'm just an ordinary person who has experimented with some age-old principles of life. They aren't really secret, yet they are not widely known, because most people are not interested in putting forth much focused effort in life. It seems like work to them, when in reality, it makes everything much easier. I have proven it to myself over and over!

I use my imagination to make work easier by seeing myself accomplishing my goals in a relaxed, comfortable manner. I imagine a project I have to do, such as writing this book. Then I focus on a key image of completion on the date I have set for it to be done. The more I focus, the easier the writing flows. Stories and examples pop up just when I need them, my schedule clears each morning for writing, and my dreams remind me of important points I want to share with you.

Getting to the Core Issue Means Improving Your Self-Image

Improving any area in life begins with modifying your self-image so it can encompass the imagined new reality. Life works most effortlessly from the inside out. By that I mean, what you feel inside about yourself is what your life will mirror back to you. Until I saw myself as someone who had a nice, new car, I couldn't get a nice, new car. Until I saw myself as someone who lived in a beautiful, clean, new setting, I could not get there.

Louise always thought of herself as an accountant, and therefore stayed an accountant. She realized more and more every year (probably right around tax season!) that she was very unhappy with her job and her life. She wanted something more in life. She wanted to be happy with her life's work, feeling that it gave her pleasure by giving others joy as well. She had been to numerous recovery groups for co-dependents and realized she could help people like herself to get over chemical dependency.

Her first goal was to believe she could change her life in this way. She began to think of herself differently. She was now a "communicator" rather than a "number cruncher." She looked into a wealth of careers in therapy and communications. If she had not changed her self-image, she would not have even known they existed. She has now embarked on a career as a therapist.

Barbara suffered from a variety of illnesses. As she became more aware of her inner workings, she realized she'd created her sickness to get attention from others. Barbara needed the love and affection the illness brought, so she kept thinking of herself as ill. But now she was ready for a change, as evidenced by her attendance in one of my classes. The more she learned about thinking thin, the more she realized that instead of just thinking fat, she had also been imagining being ill all of her life.

As she refocused her imagination on wellness, Barbara began to see a dramatic change in her health. Now she experimented with the same principles to accept the health that was trying to reach her. Barbara has simply widened her focus so she can now receive the things in life that were blocked by her previously limited imagination.

"I got really tired of accepting other people's diagnosis of me, after having gone to many doctors. I had gone to one doctor who diagnosed me as having Epstein-Barr Virus. I was just really tired of spending all my money on health products and all my time on seeing myself in an unhealthy way. The principles of thinking thin helped me see that my unhealthy self-image was being manifested by my subconscious.

"As I studied my life, I realized that time and again I would imagine myself with a particular disorder— and that would be exactly what I was dealing with. I was creating it in my body. Your book validated what I was actually experiencing, so I just used the power of imagination to imagine a new, healthy self.

"I also had to learn how not to agree with other people's thoughts, because everybody in my family saw me as sickly. That turned out to be the hardest part of the process. Sometimes it was very subtle how someone was envisioning me or the type of agreements I would enter into with other people about my health.

"I uncovered familiar patterns of playing victim and saying, 'Oh poor me.' I even realized that one powerful reason for creating my illnesses was that nobody would expect more from me than I could handle.

"An incredible healing began for me as I started to work with the principles in *How to Think Yourself Thin*. The techniques helped me uncover the destructive images I was hiding from myself. My healing was very dramatic. I began thinking myself healthy, and I was healthy.

"And here's a real key: Even though I could still see certain symptoms, I would just cancel them out of my self-image and go on. I never had a day when I wasn't working toward a better image of myself. I my kept goals in mind and pretty soon I was completely lacking the symptoms of my diagnosed illness— something which should have landed me in bed for three years according to other people's thoughts.

"Then I began replacing the real root of my illness— a thought form that said: I'm kind of crippled, so you can't expect or force me to do anything. I am still working on that one. Sometimes my mind still says, I don't have to work too hard because I'm an invalid.

"I've had some pretty funny things happen. Recently a friend wanted to come stay with me. My apartment needed a thorough cleaning, so I called a cleaning service. When they didn't show up, I thought: *Oh no! Now I have to tell my friend she can't stay here.* Then I caught myself in the act. I was startled to hear my next thought: *I'm an invalid, so I can't clean the house by myself.* I decided right then and there to change that image of myself, so I hopped up and got to work. Within four hours I was feeling fine and the apartment was ready for guests!

"I used to just look at someone sneezing at work and go home sneezing too. Although we are much more than our thoughts, the subconscious really does manifest what we think. When you make an agreement with something by thinking: *Uh huh, that will happen to me,* it's like walking into a room and saying: *'I live here.'* That becomes your reality until you want to step out of that room and live somewhere better."

Jane's experiences reflect what holds true for any statement, thought or image we have about ourselves. I have to watch myself all the time. If I say, *"I'm so tired"* a lot, I find myself feeling much more tired than if I focus on being energetic and look for ways to increase my energy.

What areas of self image would you like to change? How would you like to improve your memory, ability to be creative, self-motivation, or anything else?

Something You Can Do Now:

1. Write here or in your journal what you would like most to change first about your self-image. You can choose from these areas if you like: How you look, feel, act, or appear to yourself and others; the thoughts you think about yourself and others; your self-confidence and openness to give and receive love; the ability to be happy and fulfilled— all by yourself; or the freedom to go your own way in life:

_____

2. Describe what form your new self-image will take in terms of changing your life.

_____

3. Create a key image for your new self-image. For example, let's say you are going to be more assertive. See yourself saying, "Let me think about it," to someone who asks you a favor you would normally say "yes" to, even though you would rather not. Remember to use all the senses when creating your key image. Put some feeling into it as well. Describe this new scenario.

_____

4. Create a key phrase for your new self-image. For example, if you are becoming a better listener, you can

say something like, *"I listen closely, with an open mind and heart."*

The Ultimate Secret Behind Thinking Thin is Knowing Who You Are

Most people who diet and gain all the weight right back are unable to see themselves thin right now. You *are* now able to see yourself thin, or you wouldn't even be reading this book! You are able to become whatever you wish to become through your imagination, which is controlled by the real you.

Who *is* the real you? What part of you is in complete control of all the other parts whenever it wants to be, giving the commands, reigning over the thoughts, feelings, and senses, which bring about our circumstances in life? It is not your mind, because that is, or should be, the servant to the real you. It is not the subconscious mind, because it simply carries out the commands of the conscious mind and your unconscious images. However, when the real self is "asleep", that is, unaware of its rightful place and position, the subconscious becomes very powerful.

No, your "real self" has been called by many names throughout the centuries and eons of time. It has been called the "divine self," the "essence," the "higher self," the "ka" by the Egyptians, and as we may be most familiar with it, the Soul.

Whatever you choose to call this "inner self" or the real you, it has the ability to control the mind, the subconscious mind, the emotions, and the physical body. It's tool is the conscious use of the imagination. Soul truly is you, the real you. It can take control of your life as you become aware of yourself in this light. Then all the other aspects of your self fall into line.

So you are more than your body, mind, and emotions. You are more than pure thought or energy. You are a magical being called "Soul". You do not have a soul, because you *are* Soul! You can prove this to yourself right now.

Something You Can Do Now:

1. Close your eyes (after you read this whole exercise!) and create a movie screen onto which you can project pictures.

2. Look at a picture of a horse. Make her walk, run, and leap over a fence.

Since your eyes were not open, you were not watching this horse with your eyes. What part of you was watching? Was it the mind? No, the mind was conjuring up the images, but it wasn't watching the pictures.

The neutral observer of all the pictures in your world is the real you, Soul. That is also the part that controls you from the highest perspective when you let it. When you are relaxed, at peace and in a state of joy, Soul is in control.

When you feel tense, anxious or panicked, the mind or emotions are running wild. Soul then simply sits back and observes, waiting for the lower emotions to finally give up and return to balance.

Your imagination is ultimately controlled by the real self, or Soul. You can use this awareness that you are Soul to create a different self-image and a better life for yourself. The times I feel most in touch with myself as Soul are when I am relaxed, calm, and peaceful inside. Decisions made from this state are usually better for me and others. If I am feeling very reactive emotionally, I try not to make any decisions, because I know they will be colored by my imbalance. The imagination can run wild from emotional energy which is not from Soul.

Would you like to become more aware of yourself as Soul? Here is an exercise that will help you get in touch with the highest view of life, from Soul, whenever you want to.

Something You Can Do:

1. Use your favorite method to relax. You can use one of the relaxation exercises in Chapter 5 if you wish.

2. Think about the time you felt the most loved. This is important to open your heart to yourself as Soul.

3. Close your eyes and imagine you are at your favorite nature spot. Feel the air and the sun on your body. See the clouds drifting overhead or hear the wind rustle through the trees. Perhaps you are on the beach and can smell the salt air. Check in with all your senses.

4. Now imagine yourself beginning to drift up to one of the clouds overhead and fly right through it. Look below at your favorite spot as it becomes smaller and smaller.

5. Think of God in whatever way you prefer, or of your spiritual teacher, guide, or guardian angel. Feel the love they have for you.

You are now completely in the viewpoint and awareness of yourself as Soul.

How do you feel in this viewpoint? Write your impressions here, or in your journal:

_____

The real secret to controlling your own life comes from being aware that you are Soul and that you can be happier by staying in that viewpoint as much as possible.

Chapter 11

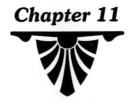

Your Thinking Thin Journal

"Recall it as often as you wish, a happy memory never wears out."
— Libbie Fudim

This chapter is your personal journal which can be used to chart your progress to realizing your new self. It can give you hope when you need a boost. It can show you just how far you have come, and provide quick reference to your own special key images and phrases.

After you have reached your first goal by thinking thin, you can return to this chapter to continue your maintenance and self-improvement.

If you would prefer not to write directly in the book, use this format as a model for your own Thinking Thin Journal. Journals are a very powerful means to understand your image process as well as motivate yourself to continue. Whenever I write in my journal, it clarifies what my next step is, what may be blocking me, and how I feel about the process. It also gets me excited as I see results through my writing.

For example, if I am feeling upset over something, I write it down. Then I keep writing until I understand what is going on inside me. It helps me to cool off and calm down so I can see the real issue. Then I may begin to write the solution. The more I write, the more enthusiastic I get about my own self-discoveries.

A few hours or even a few days later, I can look back at what I have written and see how much I have changed. It amazes me!

I also use my journal to write down dreams and questions I would like answered in my dreams. Another use of my journal is simply writing to God. If I am really stumped about something, I ask a question. If I am really happy about something, I write a thank you note! You can be as creative as you like with your journal. What I have set up for you here can be very helpful if you choose to use it.

How to Use This Journal For Maximum Benefit

As you begin the process of thinking thin, read or write something in your journal every single day. After you feel you are breaking ground, come back to it at least weekly to revise your images and thoughts about yourself and expand upon your new unlimited viewpoint.

When you have almost reached your goal, come back to the journal again to recognize and appreciate your progress, so you will maintain it. Celebrate and acknowledge your achievement. Then immediately establish new goals to keep moving forward.

Something You Can Do Now:

Take a moment right now to block out a specific time of day, preferably when you are doing your thinking thin exercises, to read and write in your journal.

I have an appointment with myself at _____.

By setting aside a specific time, your mind will willingly comply and open the gates of creativity and imagination when you sit down to write. Remember, the mind loves patterns and will eventually nag you if you miss your appointment to think thin.

Date each entry in your journal so you can see the progress you are making and how very quickly!

Becoming Childlike and Open With Yourself Will Get You Off to a Good Start

Here's a drawing exercise that you can do to bring out your childlike nature and open up your creativity. Even if you don't think you can draw, try it anyway and do the best you can. It is for your eyes only!

Something You Can Do:

In the space below, draw a picture of yourself as you would like to look. Remember that this is just for fun and to help you develop your imaginative abilities. If you would rather not draw, find a picture in a magazine of a body you would like to have now and paste your head on it.

You could also use a picture of yourself from the past that you really like. Paste it here or somewhere you will see it often. I found an old picture of myself from high school that looked really slim and put it on my refrigerator. I left it there even after I had thought myself thin, for easier maintenance.

Refer to this picture when you want to remind yourself of your new self-image.

Changing Your Self-Image is the Key to Changing Your Life

Seeing yourself *now* as you want to be in the future is paramount to success. Use your journal to really delve into this area and develop the feeling of the new you. You want to make it so real to yourself that it becomes your present reality, moving aside all other perceptions of yourself.

Instructions: Use the heading I've supplied to begin writing your key images and ideals. Do this daily for the first week. Add to them each time you reread your journal after that— at least once a week. Each heading has been allotted an entire page because you will always think of more details to add. As you date each entry, you will see how far you have come in your ability to see yourself in a new way. The more successes you see, the more courageous you will be about noting what you want to change.

Remember to write your key image in the present tense, as if you were "acting the part" of your new self. For example, "My body is more than slim, but also firm and youthful looking." You can include details of what clothes you now wear, how easily you move, how much healthier and energetic you feel, and how others react to you.

How I Look:

_____

How I Feel:

_____

How I Think About Myself:

_____

How I Act:

_____

Develop Key Images and Key Phrases For Everything You Want to Change

Remember to use all your senses as you write. What are you doing? What do you see, taste, hear, smell, and feel? Use only positives for your key phrases. For example, "I feel happy, contented, at peace."

Modify your entries to meet your new self-image each time you see beyond your present horizon. Use the "date" spaces to enter the date each time you upgrade your image.

Key Image and Key Phrase for How I Look:
Date each one as you upgrade it.

Date:_____

_____

_____

Date:_____

_____

_____

Date:_____

_____

_____

Key Image and Key Phrase For How I Feel:

Date:_____

_____

_____

Date:_____

_____

_____

Date:_____

_____

_____

Key Image and Phrase For How I Act:

Date:_____

_____

_____

Date:_____

_____

_____

Date:_____

_____

_____

Key Image For How I Think About Myself:

Date:_____

_____

_____

Date:_____

_____

_____

Date:_____

_____

_____

Dream Journal

Use this section to ask for and record dreams that re-
late to changing your self-image. Record and date your
specific question, and the corresponding dreams. Then
brainstorm on how the dream answers your question.

It is so much fun to explore the effectiveness of your
dreams. As in the Dream Exercise in Chapter 5, after
writing down the dream or pieces of a dream, write, "The
meaning of this dream is:" Then just write whatever
comes to mind.

Questions I Would Like Answered in My Dreams:

Date:_____Question:_____

_____

Answer or Dream: _____

_____

This Dream Means:

_____

Date:_____Question:_____

_____

Answer or Dream: _____

This Dream Means:

_____

Date:_____Question:_____

_____

Answer or Dream: _____

This Dream Means:

_____

You can continue to keep a record of your dreams in a notebook. Set up a dream journal especially for your dream questions and dreams. Or you can integrate your dream journal into your personal journal, as I do. I find that "life is but a dream," so I don't bother to separate my waking and sleeping life. I encounter "waking dreams" all the time that reveal my limitations and how to resolve them— if I observe very closely. Combining all my experiences help me see any patterns that are emerging day to day.

If you try this, it will become obvious to you that there is indeed a divine design to your life worth looking at. That pattern will make everything clearer and you will know what steps to take to improve your life next!

Charting Your Progress Can Be Fun and Rewarding

Here is an excellent way to begin discovering some of your life patterns. Even if you do not have time to log your dreams or can't remember them, you can still note your experiences, thoughts and feelings about life while you are taking this safari through the subconscious.

Something You Can Do Now:

For the first week of your thinking thin experiment, write daily statements about how you are thinking and feeling about yourself differently and how your health and diet-related issues are transforming.

Day # 1   Date:_____ How I feel and think:

_____

What is happening in my life:

_____

Day #2   Date:_____ How I feel and think:

_____

What is happening in my life:

_____

Day #3   Date:_____ How I feel and think:

_____

What is happening in my life:

_____

Day #4   Date:_____   How I feel and think:

_____

What is happening in my life:

_____

Day #5   Date:_____   How I feel and think:

_____

What is happening in my life:

_____

Day #6   Date:_____   How I feel and think:

_____

What is happening in my life:

_____

Day #7   Date:_____   How I feel and think:

_____

What is happening in my life:

_____

Now that you have logged your innermost feelings and outward experiences for a week, go back and read each day. What kind of progress can you see? Write it here or in your journal:

_____

Now do the same thing for the next month, writing weekly recaps of your constant progress so you will always be aware of it.

Week #1   Date:_____   How I feel and think:

_____

What is happening in my life:

_____

Week #2   Date:_____   How I feel and think:

_____

What is happening in my life:

_____

Week #3   Date:_____   How I feel and think:

_____

What is happening in my life:

_____

Week #4   Date:_____   How I feel and think:

_____

What is happening in my life:

_____

Now that you have charted your progress for a whole month, read over all four weeks. What kind of progress do you see over the past month?

Write it here or in your journal:

_____

Maintaining the New You and Continuing Your Progress Is Easy With Focus

Writing in your journal helps you to maintain your focus. Anything which has your attention has a much greater chance of succeeding. Remember, there are only two directions you can go from here; backward or forward. Which do you choose?

The simplest way to keep your attention focused forward, on the positive benefits of thinking thin, is by practicing gratitude and celebration. As you track your weekly and monthly progress, be sure to thank and reward yourself for thinking thin, a secret to long-term progress and maintenance.

Something You Can Do:

Here is an exercise to continue being grateful for your progress, however small or great it is.

On a monthly basis, for the next six months, write here what is new in your life that you are happy about and thankful for.

Month #1   Date:_____ I am grateful for:

_____

Month #2   Date:_____ I am grateful for:

_____

Month #3   Date:_____ I am grateful for:

_____

Month #4 Date:_____ I am grateful for:

_____

Month #5 Date:_____ I am grateful for:

_____

Month #6 Date:_____ I am grateful for:

_____

Now look back at months one through six. What kind of progress do you see in your life regarding thinking thin or any other successes? Write them here or in your journal:

_____

Use a notebook to continue this gratitude exercise. I like to think of my gratitude markers as love letters to God. I write them whenever I feel so filled with love and joy in my life that I just have to express it by being grateful. It brings more wonderful things into my life when I remember to do so!

What Else Would You Like to Change About Your Body or Your Life?

Remember that you can use any and all of the thinking thin exercises to change your body or your life.

Something You Can Do:

The following pages are categorized listings of the different areas people generally want to change. At the end there is an "other" section for aspects of your life which may not be listed.

As in all the other simple exercises in this journal, follow this recipe for success. 1. Develop a key image and key phrase for your new self-image. 2. Relax and focus on your image and phrase at least once a day. Remember to have fun and play at this imagination game!

What I Want For Optimum Fitness/Health/Body:

Key Image:

_____

Key Phrase:

_____

What I Want For the Optimum Intimate Relationship/ Marriage:

Key Image:

_____

Key Phrase:

_____

What I Want For the Optimum Financial Situation:

Key Image:

_____

Key Phrase:

_____

What I Want For the Optimum Career:

Key Image:

_____

Key Phrase:

_____

What I Want For the Optimum Spiritual Experience/Life:

Key Image:

_____

Key Phrase:

_____

What I Want For the Optimum Family Experience:

Key Image:

_____

Key Phrase:

_____

What I Want For the Optimum Parenting Experience:

Key Image:

_____

Key Phrase:

_____

What I want For the Optimum Friendships:

Key Image:

_____

Key Phrase:

_____

What I Want For the Optimum Home/House:

Key Image:

_____

Key Phrase:

_____

What I Want For the Optimum Creative Outlet (Music, Art, Dance, or My Hobby):

Key Image:

_____

Key Phrase:

_____

What I Want For the Optimum Continued Education:

Key Image:

_____

Key Phrase:

_____

What I Want For the Optimum

(You Fill in the Blank):

Key Image:

Key Phrase:

Chapter 12

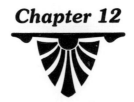

Recapturing How To Think Yourself Thin

"The food that enters the mind must be watched as closely as the food that enters the body."
— Patrick J. Buchanan

Copy these pages and carry them in your purse or briefcase. Post them at home on the mirror or refrigerator, in your car, by your bedside or wherever you feel they will benefit you the most. They are intended to be an easy reference for those who like to use the principle of focused attention to the maximum!

Use the Subconscious to Push You Forward

When you consciously control your thoughts, you can change your self-image and body. What do you want to achieve? Imagine it constantly. Pretending like a child that it is *true now.*

Accept and Love Yourself Just as You Are Now

Write your five best qualities here and read them whenever you feel your self-image is waning:

1. _____

2. _____

3. _____

4. _____

5. _____

Focus On Your Key Image
(Remember to Relax)

Write your key image for thinking thin here and focus on it daily:

_____

_____

Repeat Your Key Phrase As Much
As Possible

Write your key phrase here and repeat it often:

_____

Use these key phrases if you need a change:
"I am happy, healthy and slim!"
"People are beginning to notice my new slim body."
"I love my new slender, graceful figure!"
"The more I think thin, the more I eat, exercise, and am thin."
"Every single thing I eat makes my body beautiful and slim."

Believe Only What Your Images Inside Convey To You

It has been proven over and over again that what you are imagining right now will be what your life gives you in the future. You are in complete control through your imagination. Use it wisely.

No matter what your outer circumstances may convey, you *will* become thin by believing that *you are thin now.* Do whatever it takes to convince the mind. Every cell in your body reacts to your thoughts. How do you want them to respond?

"As a man thinketh, so is he." And of course this applies to women too!

This is a divine gift. Use it with love for yourself and in love and service to all for the greatest achievements and the greatest happiness.

Be Grateful For Every Single Bit of Progress You Make

Write love notes to God, or just say thank you inside for the progress you have made just by putting the effort forth with love. Accept every compliment as true. You *will* see results by doing so.

Highlight or Rewrite the Ideas You Need to Work On Most

Record your favorite three ideas from *How to Think Yourself Thin* here:

1. _____

2. _____

3. _____

You can also make a personal tape recording of your key image and phrase. The tape can include your favorite principles from this book. Read aloud from it or put the concepts into your own words. Listen to it right before you go to sleep, in your car, or when relaxing.

Remember Who You Are— and Have a Ball With This!

Remember that you are a glowing, loving being called Soul. No matter what happens, you have become a brighter light already, just by recognizing your own sovereignty over the mind, emotions, and physical self!

Make thinking thin as fun as you can, and you will automatically be operating from the highest perspective, that of Soul. The joyful, playful, childlike state will bring you best results. Play at imagining your key images as if it were a simple game. See how far you can go. You may be very surprised!

Suggested Reading

Books for Proof This Works:

1. *How to Become Naturally Thin by Eating More*, by Jean Antonello.

2. *Learn While You Sleep*, by David Autis.

3. *Psychopsybernetics*, by Maxwell Maltz

4. *Hidden Power: How to Unleash the Power of the Subconscious Mind*, by Van Fleet.

Other books by Debbie Johnson:

How to Love Yourself, So Others Can Love You More, $6.95.
The secret of bringing more love into your life is inside you.
Stories, methods, and specific "exercises" to bring more love into your life and to nurture yourself as well.

How to Make Your Dreams Come True, $6.95.
Discover the magic of life's simply mysteries.
Take the next step— make your whole life an adventure! In parable form, this book breaks through the impossible to move you into the probable! Last chapter is a workbook.

To Order: 1-800-444-2524

Books for Attitude and Soul Viewpoints:

1.　*The Flute of God* and other books by Paul Twitchell or Harold Kemp.

2.　*Quantum Healing* and other books by Dr. Deepak Chopra.

3.　*When You Believe It You Will See It*, and other books by Dr. Wayne Dyer.

Suggested Listening

Audio Cassettes:

1.　*Imagine Yourself Slim*, by Dr. Emmett Miller (Source Cassettes: 1-800-52tapes or bookstore).

2.　*Hu- A Love Song to God*, by Harold Kemp (Illuminated Way Publishing: 1-800-457-9063, or ask your bookstore to order from IWP).

To request **Debbie Johnson** for workshops or speaking engagements call **Deborah Johnson** Publishing at **(503) 292-7657**

Think Yourself Thin Workshop Now on Video Tape!!!

Do-it-yourself Workshop
Invite friends and family
Start your own support group (see Chapter 8)

Workshop by Debbie Johnson, author of *How to Think Yourself Thin*, was recorded in her own living room, from her home to yours, and from her heart to yours. Takes you step by step through your own body shaping process!

To order additional copies of this book, or other books by Debbie Johnson, or the "Think Yourself Thin" Video

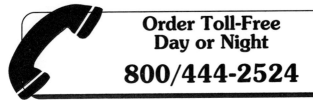

**Order Toll-Free
Day or Night
800/444-2524**